Imaging of Perianal Inflammatory Diseases

Massimo Tonolini • Giovanni Maconi
Editors

Imaging of Perianal Inflammatory Diseases

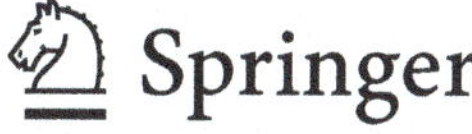

Editors
Massimo Tonolini
Radiology Department
Luigi Sacco University Hospital
Milan, Italy

Giovanni Maconi
Gastroenterology Unit
Department of Biomedical and Clinical Sciences
Luigi Sacco University Hospital
Milan, Italy

ISBN 978-88-470-2846-3 ISBN 978-88-470-2847-0 (eBook)

DOI 10.1007/978-88-470-2847-0

Springer Milan Dordrecht Heidelberg London New York
Library of Congress Control Number: 2012951704

9 8 7 6 5 4 3 2 1 2013 2014 2015 2016

Cover design: Ikona S.r.l., Milan, Italy
Typesetting: Graphostudio, Milan, Italy
Printing and binding: Arti Grafiche Nidasio S.r.l., Assago (MI), Italy

Springer-Verlag Italia S.r.l. – Via Decembrio 28 – I-20137 Milan
Springer is a part of Springer Science+Business Media (www.springer.com)

In memory of Dr. Francesco Lazzerini
and Prof. Carlo M. Uslenghi

Massimo

Preface

Imaging of the rectum, anorectal junction, and surrounding tissues has always been challenging, but in recent years magnetic resonance imaging (MRI) and ultrasound have significantly improved visualization of the anorectum and of perianal diseases. The time is therefore ripe for a book that sets out clearly the role of these imaging techniques, and also computed tomography, in the diagnosis and management of perianal inflammatory disease.

The contents of this book are based closely on the extensive experience gained at Luigi Sacco University Hospital in Milan. The principal focus is on the chronic inflammatory intestinal diseases, Crohn's disease and ulcerative colitis, and the associated perianal fistulas, but cryptogenic fistulas, sexually transmitted diseases, cancer arising in perianal fistulas, and rare diseases are also covered.

A particular feature of the book is its collaborative multidisciplinary approach deriving from the fact that the authors include gastroenterologists and surgeons as well as radiologists. Together, this multitalented team, who benefit from knowledge of each other's work, provide detailed practical information on diagnosis and management.

Readers will find descriptions of the surgical, MRI, and ultrasound anatomy of the anorectal region, up-to-date clinical and therapeutic information on the full range of perianal inflammatory conditions, and instruction on clinical examination and surgical approaches.

The main body of the book, however, is devoted to the role of ultrasound and MRI. Guidance is provided on the performance of transanal and transperineal ultrasound and on the MRI study protocol, and the value of the imaging techniques in disease classification, staging, assessment of complications, and treatment follow-up is explained in detail. Readers will also benefit from the numerous imaging examples, the identification of common artifacts and pitfalls, and the provision of a diagnostic algorithm with integration of the different imaging modalities.

It has been a pleasure to coordinate the efforts of colleagues from different specialties who have, we believe, succeeded in producing a book that will serve as a state of the art guide to the use of diagnostic imaging techniques in patients with perianal inflammatory diseases and an invaluable aid to assessment, management, and follow-up.

Milan, October 2012

Massimo Tonolini
Giovanni Maconi

Contents

Contributors

Sandro Ardizzone Gastroenterology Unit, Department of Biomedical and Clinical Sciences, Luigi Sacco University Hospital, Milan, Italy

Guido Basilisco Gastroenterology Unit, IRCCS Cà Granda Ospedale Maggiore Policlinico, Milan, Italy

Giulia Bella Radiologic, Oncologic and Anatomopathological Sciences, Policlinico Umberto I, Rome, Italy

Cristina Bezzio Gastroenterology Unit, Department of Biomedical and Clinical Sciences, Luigi Sacco University Hospital, Milan, Italy

Elena Bolzacchini Gastroenterology Unit, Department of Biomedical and Clinical Sciences, Luigi Sacco University Hospital, Milan, Italy

Andrea Bondurri General Surgery 1, Luigi Sacco University Hospital, Milan, Italy

Valeria Buonocore Radiologic, Oncologic and Anatomopathological Sciences, Policlinico Umberto I, Rome, Italy

Alessandro Campari Diagnostic and Interventional Radiology Department, San Paolo Hospital – University of Milan, Milan, Italy

Flavio Caprioli Surgical Physiopathology and Transplants, University of Milan, Milan, Italy

Andrea Cassinotti Gastroenterology Unit, Luigi Sacco University Hospital, Milan, Italy

Francesco Colombo Department of Surgery, Gastroenterology and Oncology, Luigi Sacco University Hospital, Milan, Italy

Gian Paolo Cornalba Diagnostic and Interventional Radiology, San Paolo Hospital, Milan, Italy

Michele Crespi Department of Surgery, Gastroenterology and Oncology, Luigi Sacco University Hospital, Milan, Italy

Piergiorgio Danelli General Surgery 1, Luigi Sacco University Hospital, Milan, Italy

Diego Foschi Department of Surgery, Gastroenterology and Oncology, Luigi Sacco University Hospital, Milan, Italy

Alice Frontali Department of Surgery, Gastroenterology and Oncology, Luigi Sacco University Hospital, Milan, Italy

Federica Furfaro Gastroenterology Unit, Department of Biomedical and Clinical Sciences, Luigi Sacco University Hospital, Milan, Italy

Francesca Maccioni Radiologic, Oncologic and Anatomopathological Sciences, Policlinico Umberto I, Rome, Italy

Giovanni Maconi Gastroenterology Unit, Department of Biomedical and Clinical Sciences, Luigi Sacco University Hospital, Milan, Italy

Matteo Marone Medicine and Surgery, University of Milan, Milan, Italy

Alice Munari Diagnostic and Interventional Radiology, San Paolo Hospital, Milan, Italy

Alba H. Norsa Radiology Department, IGEA Clinic, Milan, Italy

Giovanni Guido Pompili Diagnostic and Interventional Radiology, San Paolo Hospital, Milan, Italy

Elisa Radice Division of Gastroenterology, University Vita e Salute San Raffaele, San Raffaele Hospital, Milan, Italy

Paolo Rigamonti Diagnostic and Interventional Radiology, San Paolo Hospital, Milan, Italy

Gianluca M. Sampietro Department of Surgery, Gastroenterology and Oncology, Luigi Sacco University Hospital, Milan, Italy

Giulio A. Santoro Head, Pelvic Floor and Colorectal Service, First Department of General Surgery, Regional Hospital, Treviso, Italy

Massimo Tonolini Radiology Department, Luigi Sacco University Hospital, Milan, Italy

Chiara Villa Radiology Department, Luigi Sacco University Hospital, Milan, Italy

Section I

Introduction

Perineum: Surgical Anatomy and Physiology

1

Andrea Bondurri, Piergiorgio Danelli and Matteo Marone

1.1 Introduction

The perineum (Fig. 1.1) is defined as the inferior outlet of the pelvis. It is a diamond-shaped area with its major axis between the pubis and the tip of the coccyx and its minor axis along the ischial tuberosity. The perineum is commonly divided into two anatomic triangles: the anterior urogenital triangle and the posterior anal triangle. The deep borders of the perineum are composed of the pubic arch, the arcuate ligament of the pubis, and, on either side, the inferior portions of the pubis and ischium.

The muscle layer comprising the pelvic diaphragm creates the "roof" of the perineum. It is composed of the levator ani and coccygeal muscles and it separates the pelvic cavity from the perineal region. The levator ani consists of three muscles: the pubococcygeus, puborectalis, and iliococcygeus. The pubococcygeus is the primary muscle; it runs backward from the pubis toward the coccyx, with some of its fibers inserted into the urethra, prostate, and vagina. The puborectalis runs from the pubis to the rectum, forming a muscular ring hardly separable from the external anal sphincter. The iliococcygeus, which makes up the posterior part of the levator ani, is often poorly developed. The coccygeal muscle, situated behind the levator ani, is frequently more tendinous than muscular. It extends from the ischial spine to the lateral margin of the sacrum and coccyx.

The base of the perineum is composed of the skin, which is tough and mobile near the intergluteal line and less mobile near the anal orifice, and the subcutaneous tissue, which is less represented close to the anal orifice [1].

A. Bondurri (✉)
General Surgery 1, Luigi Sacco University Hospital
Milan, Italy
e-mail: bondurri.andrea@hsacco.it

M.Tonolini and G. Maconi (eds.), *Imaging of Perianal Inflammatory Diseases*,
DOI: 10.1007/978-88-470-2847-0_1, © Springer-Verlag Italia 2013

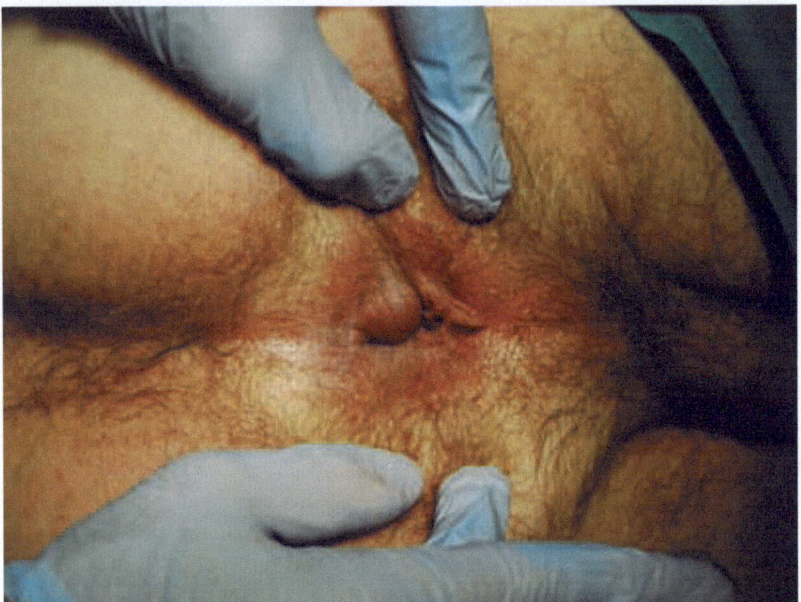

Fig. 1.1 The perineum

Dissecting the skin layer reveals the external anal sphincter and between it and the lateral border of the perineum the ischioanal fossa. This fossa has a prismatic shape, with its base directed towards the surface of the perineum and its apex meeting the obturator and anal fasciae. The lateral border is composed of the obturator internus muscle and its fascia. The pudendal vessels and nerves are located in a splitting of this latter fascia. The medial border is formed by the levator ani and the external anal sphincter. The ischioanal fossa has two extensions, an anterior one between the levator ani and perineal fascia, and a posterior one, between the levator ani and gluteus major [3].

1.2 The Urogenital Triangle

The musculotendinous layer of the urogenital triangle closes the anterior part of the pelvis. In males, it is crossed by the urethra and bulbo-urethral glands, and in females by the urethra, vagina, and vestibular glands. It is composed of several different layers: the deep transverse perineal muscle, between the bones of the ischium; the urethral sphincter surrounding the urethra; the ischiocavernosus muscle, extending from the inner surface of the ischial tuberosity to the pubic bones; and a bulbospongiosus muscle arising from the central tendinous point of the perineum. In males, it encircles the urethra and in females it covers the vestibular bulb and envelops the vagina [1].

1.3 The Anal Triangle

The most important structure of the anal triangle is of course the anal canal. Developmentally, it is a region of fusion between endodermal and ectodermal tubes, evident at the dentate line. The distal colon is derived from the hindgut and is thus made up of endodermal tissue. Before the 5th gestational week, the intestinal and urogenital tract flow in the cloaca. During the 6th gestational week, the two tracts separate. The anal canal is the terminal portion of the large intestine. It forms an angle with the lower part of the rectum, measures 2.5–4 cm, and is surrounded by the internal and external anal sphincters. A variable number of vertical folds, the rectal columns, lie 7–15 mm above the anal orifice and are separated from each other by rectal sinuses, which end in the anal valves.

The anorectal blood supply comes from the superior and inferior hemorrhoidal arteries, which in turn derive, respectively, from the superior mesenteric and pudendal arteries. The veins of the rectum and anal canal converge in a plexus that surrounds the canal and contains small saccular dilatations just within the margin of the anus. This plexus typically gives off six vessels of considerable size that penetrate the muscular coat and converge in a single trunk, the superior hemorrhoidal vein. This so-called hemorrhoidal plexus communicates with the tributaries of the middle and inferior hemorrhoidal veins and establishes a communication between the systemic and portal circulations.

The muscular structure of the anal canal is composed of the external and internal sphincter ani. The external sphincter measures 8–10 cm in length and about 2.5 cm in width. Its elliptical muscular fibers are intimately adherent to the margin of the anus. Of the two layers that comprise the external anal sphincter, the lateral layer, formed by fibers from the levator ani muscle, is the main one. The deep layer forms a complete sphincter surrounding the anal canal and it is closely applied to the internal anal sphincter. It is always in a state of tonic contraction and has no antagonistic muscle, which allows it to keep the anal canal and orifice closed. According to will, it can be put in a state of more firm contraction to occlude anal opening.

The internal anal sphincter is a muscular ring that surrounds the anal canal. It is about 5 mm thick and is formed by an aggregation of involuntary circular muscular fibers. Between the two sphincters is the intersphincteric space, which is important in the pathogenesis of perianal abscesses because it contains most of the anal glands.

Motor innervation of the rectum is provided by sympathetic and parasympathetic nerves. The external anal sphincter is innervated by the inferior rectal branch of the pudendal nerve (S3 S4) and by the perineal branch of S4. Sensory innervation is provided by free nerve terminations as well as organized nerve endings and derives from the inferior rectal branch of the pudendal nerve [1-3].

1.4 Defecation

The anorectum (Fig. 1.2) acts as a reservoir, with a capacity of about 0.5 l, and as a "pump" for the evacuation of feces. Defecation involves the semi-voluntary emptying of the rectum and requires a sequence of events that integrates smooth and striated muscle and the central, somatic, autonomic, and enteric nervous systems.

Defecation begins with rectal distension caused by caudally migrating contractions that originate in the colon and drive feces from there to the rectum. When a characteristic threshold is reached, an awareness of rectal filling begins. The intensity of this sensation increases as the rectum continues to fill until it becomes an urge to defecate. Distension of the rectum causes various reflexes that end in the contraction of the rectum itself, relaxation of the internal anal sphincter, and contraction of the external anal sphincter. During defecation, the anal canal must be open and the intrarectal pressure must exceed the anal canal pressure. Straightening of the anorectal angle and, subsequently, opening of the rectum require that contraction of the pelvic floor is inhibited. The pelvic floor descends and muscle contraction shortens the anal canal. In a Valsalva maneuver, intrarectal pressure increases, assisting defecation. Defecation terminates when contraction of the puborectalis and external anal

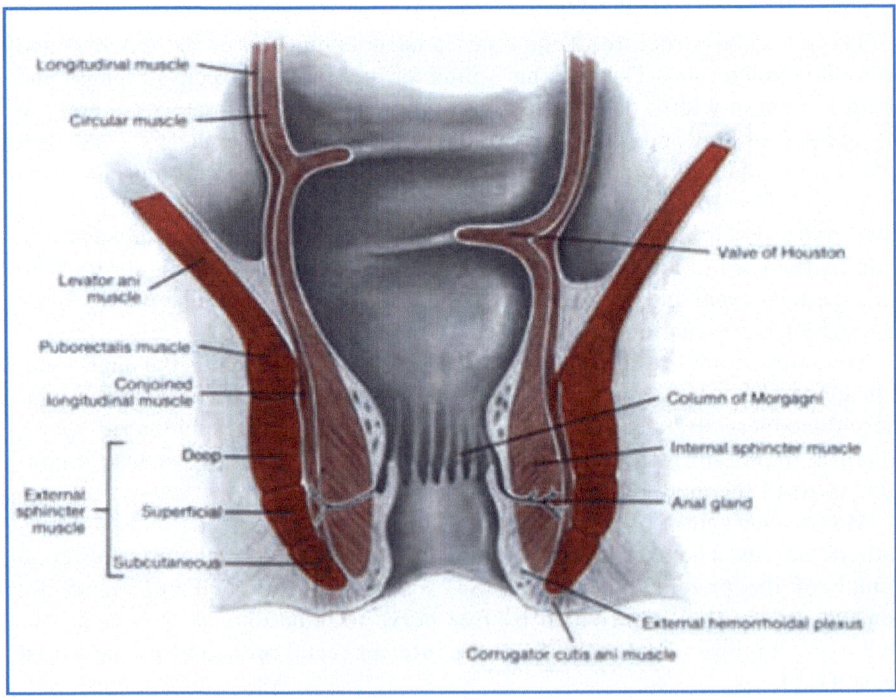

Fig. 1.2 Transverse view of the anorectum

sphincter restores the anorectal angle, the internal anal sphincter recovers its tone, and the anal canal closes [4].

References

1. Balboni G (2007) Trattato di anatomia umana, 4th edn. Edi Ermes, Milan, pp. 122-134, 467-472
2. Towsend CBR, Evers B (2008) Sabiston text book of surgery: the biological basis of modern surgical practice, 18th edn. Saunders Elsevier, Philadelphia, pp. 1447–1449
3. Corman ML (2005) Colon& rectal surgery, 5th edn. Lippincot Williams & Wilkins, Philadelphia, pp. 7-27, 279-332
4. Brookes, SJ, Dinning PG, Gladman MA (2009) Neuroanatomy and physiology of colorectal function and defaecation: from basic science to human clinical studies. Neurogastroenterol Motil. 21(2):9-19

MRI Anatomy of the Anorectal Region

2

Giovanni Guido Pompili, Alice Munari, Paolo Rigamonti
and Gian Paolo Cornalba

2.1 Anatomy

The anatomy of the perianal region can be accurately demonstrated with magnetic resonance imaging (MRI). The anal canal begins at the level of the levator ani and extends until the anus, resulting in a typical length of 2.5–5 cm. It is surrounded by the internal and external anal sphincters. The puborectalis muscle forms the top of the anorectal ring and continues caudally in the joined longitudinal muscles and subsequently in the external anal sphincter muscle.

The following is a brief description of the specific imaging terms used for pelvic floor structures with reference to imaging planes.

Internal anal sphincter (IAS). This is a well-defined ring of smooth muscle fibers that are an extension of the circular layer of the muscularis propria of the rectum. The IAS is enveloped superiorly by the levator ani muscle and distally by the superficial portion of the external sphincter muscle and subsequently by its subcutaneous portion. It stops approximately 1 cm above the lower edge of the external anal sphincter. As an involuntary sphincter, the IAS is responsible for 85% of resting anal tone. In most patients, it can be surgically divided without causing a loss of continence (Fig. 2.1).

Anal smooth muscle (ASM). The two muscles that form the ASM, the longitudinal rectal muscle (LRM) and its caudal extension, the IAS (Fig. 2.1), cannot be individually distinguished on the basis of MRI.

Intersphincteric space (ISS). Within this space are all structures between the ASM and external anal sphincter. The ISS is divided into outer and inner components by the joint longitudinal muscle, which is formed by the extension

G.G. Pompili (✉)
Diagnostic and Interventional Radiology, San Paolo Hospital
Milan, Italy
e-mail: gpompili@sirm.org

M.Tonolini and G. Maconi (eds.), *Imaging of Perianal Inflammatory Diseases*,
DOI: 10.1007/978-88-470-2847-0_2, © Springer-Verlag Italia 2013

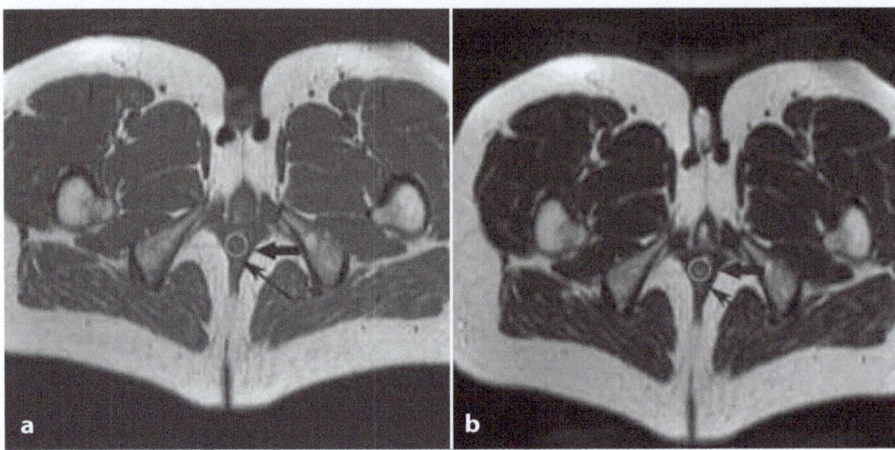

Fig. 2.1 **a** Axial T1-weighted image. **b** Axial T2-weighted image shows the complex of internal and external anal sphincters: IAS (*circle*), ISS (*thin arrow*), and EAS (*thick arrow*)

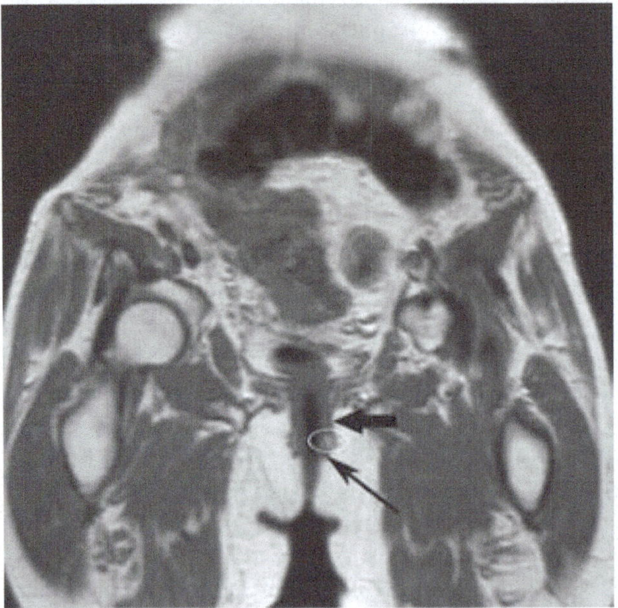

Fig. 2.2 Coronal T1-weighted image. The three different portions of the EAS: deep (*thick arrow*), subcutaneous (*circle*), and superficial (*thin arrow*)

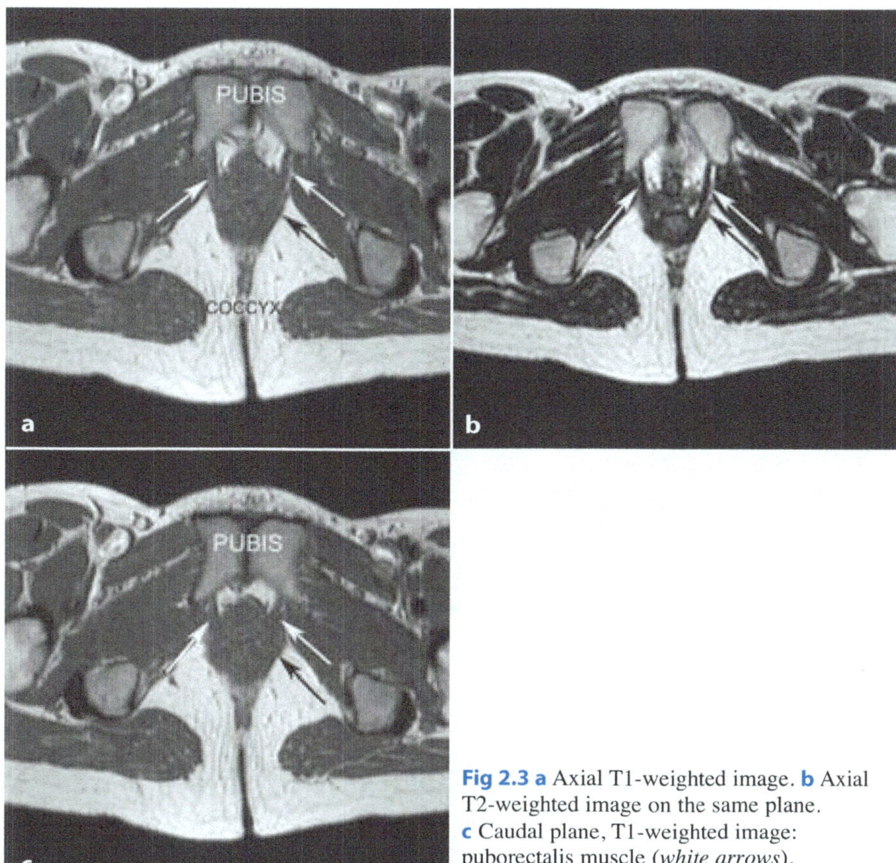

Fig 2.3 a Axial T1-weighted image. **b** Axial T2-weighted image on the same plane. **c** Caudal plane, T1-weighted image: puborectalis muscle (*white arrows*), pubococcygeal muscle (*black arrow*)

of the smooth longitudinal layer of the rectum and the vertical portion of the elevator ani, particularly the puboanalis. The ISS measures 2–7 mm in men and 2–5 mm in women and it is contiguous with the upper supralevator space. Both the inner and the outer ISS have high signal intensity on T1 and T2, determined by their fatty composition (Fig. 2.1).

External anal sphincter (EAS). The striated muscle of the EAS continues superiorly to form the levator ani and the puborectalis. The EAS can be divided craniocaudally in three parts: deep, superficial, and subcutaneous (Fig. 2.2; see also Fig. 2.11). The middle third of the EAS surrounds the inferior portion of the IAS and is connected anteriorly to the tendinous center of the perineum and posteriorly to the anococcygeal ligament. While the EAS maintains only 15% of resting anal tone, its strong voluntary contraction is fundamental for defecation. Surgical division of the EAS can lead to incontinence.

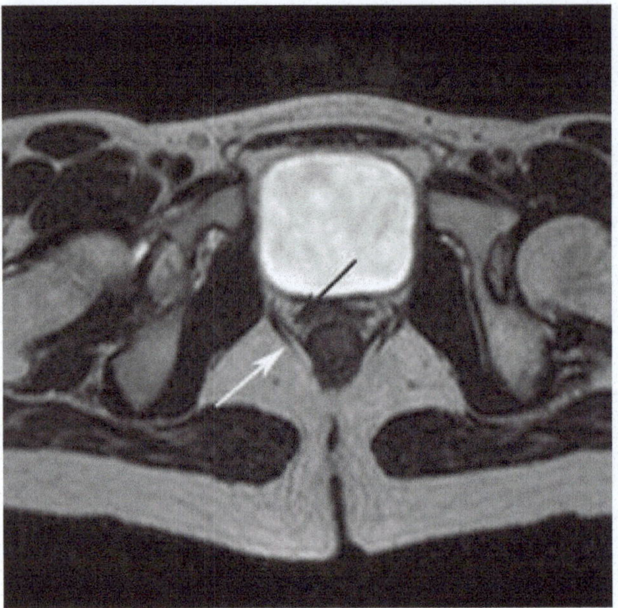

Fig. 2.4 Axial T2-weighted image. Pubococcygeal muscle (*black arrow*), iliococcygeal muscle (*white arrow*)

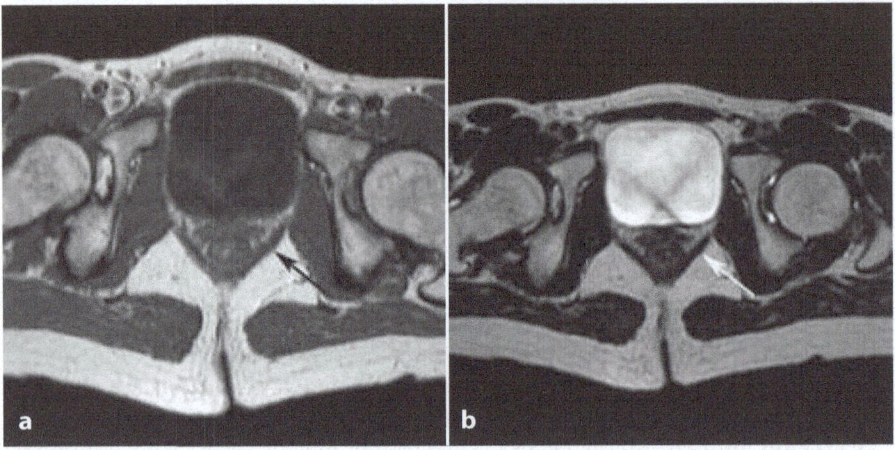

Fig. 2.5 **a** Axial T1-weighted image. **b** Axial T2-weighted image: iliococcygeal muscle (*arrow*)

Levator ani. The three muscles that form the levator ani are, from medial to lateral: the **puborectalis** (Fig. 2.3a–c), the **pubococcygeal** (Figs. 2.3, 2.4 and 2.6), and the **iliococcygeal** (Figs. 2.4–2.6). They support the viscera of the pelvic cavity, coordinate defecation-related functions, and join the coccygeal muscle to

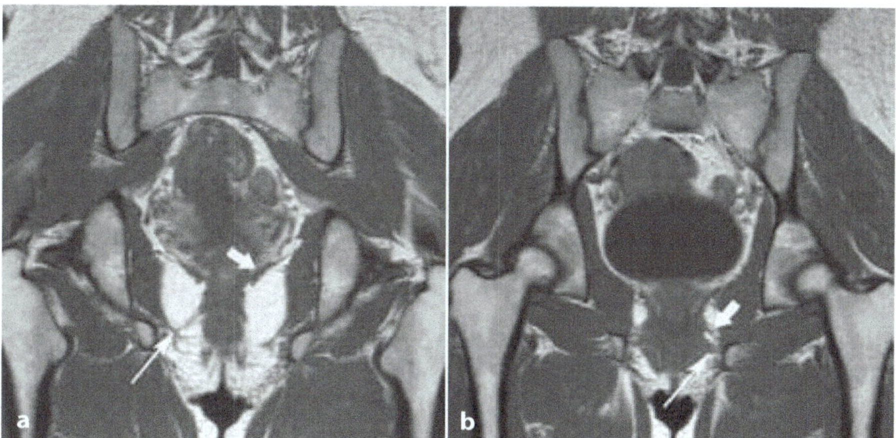

Fig. 2.6 Coronal T1-weighted image. **a** Dorsal plane: iliococcygeal muscle (*thick arrow*), pubococcygeal muscle (*thin arrow*). **b** Ventral plane: puborectalis muscle (*thick arrow*), superficial transverse perineal muscle (*thin arrow*)

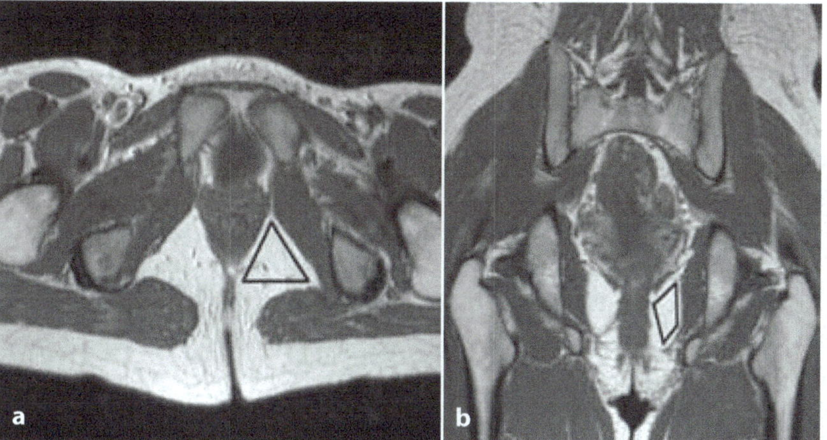

Fig. 2.7 Ischioanal space shown on an axial T1-weighted image (*triangle* in **a**) and coronal T1-weighted image (*diamond* in **b**)

form the pelvic diaphragm. The puborectalis muscle begins at the back of the pubis and from the top end of the urogenital diaphragm, continuing posteriorly on the contralateral side to form a U-shaped puborectal sling, located at the anorectal junction. Subsequently, it is connected with the deep layer of the EAS. The **puboperinealis** is the anterolateral continuation of the puborectalis; it has a rounded triangular shape and is closely related to the bladder floor and the membranous urethra.

Ischioanal space (IA). Triangular in shape, it lies laterally to the EAS and caudally to the levator ani muscle (Fig. 2.7a, b).

Perineal body. This structure is larger in women than in men because it protects the EAS during childbirth. Also in women, it separates anatomical structures located between the posterior distal wall of the vagina and the anterior anal canal. In men, the perineal body is not well visible because it is strictly connected to the EAS and to the perineal muscles (Fig. 2.8).

Superficial transverse perineal muscles. On the axial plane, this muscle is well-visualized as a wide and thin muscular layer cranial to the anterior EAS and connected to the perineal body. In the coronal plane, the left and right superficial transverse perineal muscles are separated medially by the bulbospongiosus muscle and insert laterally into the fascia of the ischiocavernous muscle. These muscles serve as the bony anchor for all perineal structures (Figs. 2.6, 2.8; also see Fig. 2.12).

Anococcygeal ligament. A ventral layer extends from the sacral fascia to the common longitudinal layer of the anal canal, while a dorsal layer extends between the coccyx and the EAS (Figs. 2.9, 2.10).

Superficial postanal space. This is the most caudal space, located posteriorly behind the end of the coccyx and under the anococcygeal ligament (Fig. 2.10).

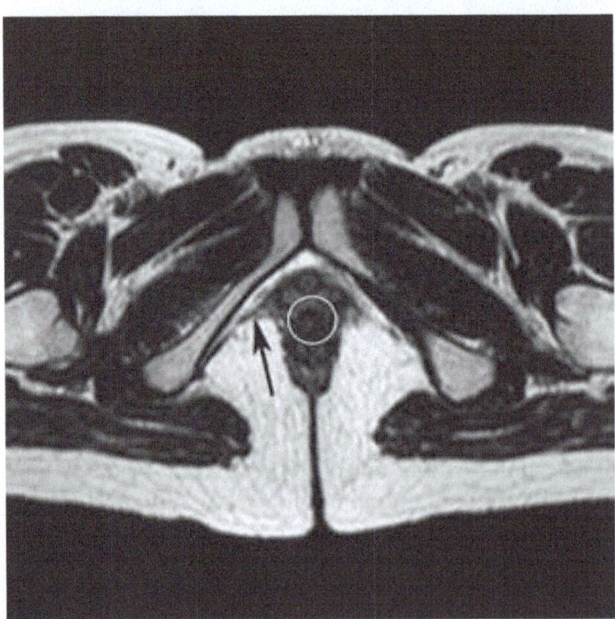

Fig. 2.8 Axial T2-weighted image. Perineal body (*circle*), superficial transverse perineal muscle (*arrow*)

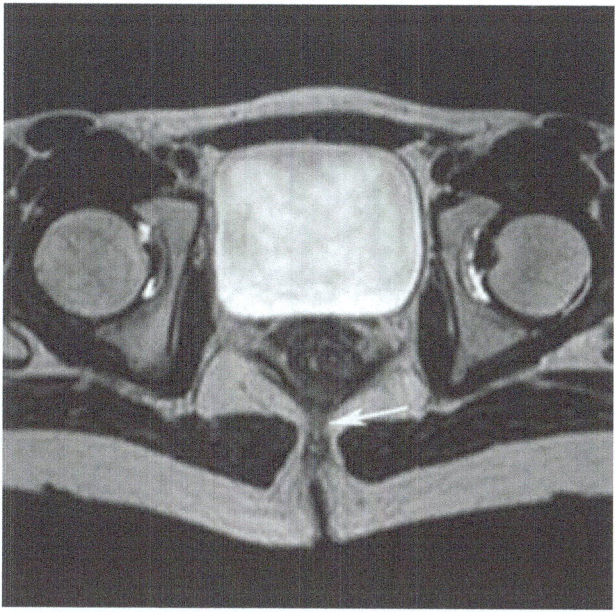

Fig. 2.9 Axial T2-weighted image. Anococcygeal ligament (*arrow*)

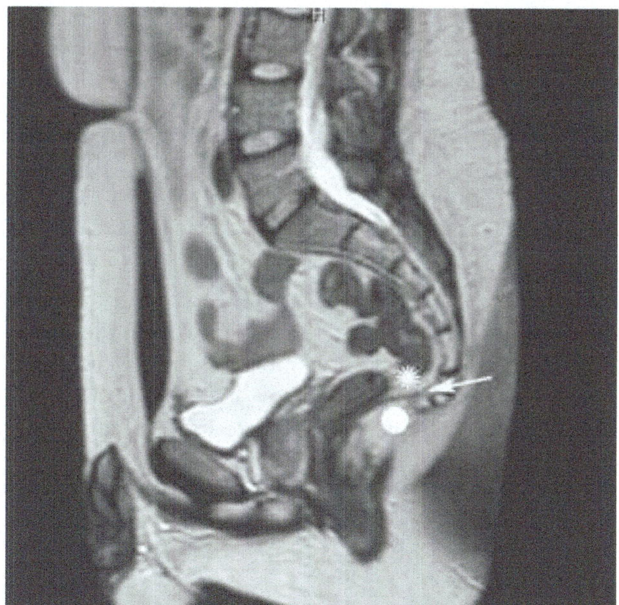

Fig. 2.10 Sagittal T2-weighted image. Anococcygeal ligament (*arrow*) and the deep (*asterisk*), and superficial (*white dot*) portions of the postanal space

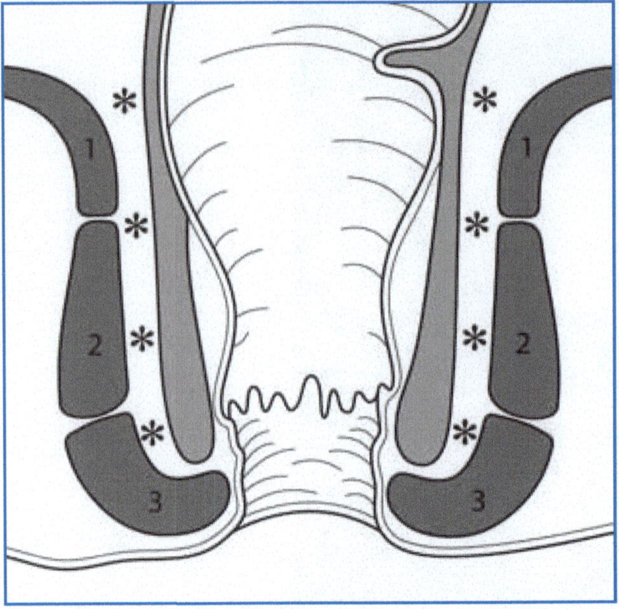

Fig. 2.11 Mid-coronal anal section: IAS (*light gray*); EAS (*dark gray*) with its three different portions: deep (*1*), subcutaneous (*2*), and superficial (*3*); intersphincteric space (*asterisks*)

Deep postanal space. This space is located below the levator ani and deep to the anococcygeal ligament. It continues laterally with the ischioanal spaces (Fig. 2.10).

Anal subcutaneous angle. This is the angle between the anus and the subcutaneous sphincter axis.

2.2 MRI Technique and Image Analysis

The different signal intensities on T1- and T2-weighted images form the basis of the imaging investigation. The mucosa, smooth muscle, striated muscle, tendons, and fibrous tissue are distinguished by their low or low-intermediate signal intensities (black), the submucosa by its intermediate-high signal intensity (gray), and fat tissue by its high signal intensity (white).

Mid-coronal anal T1- and T2-weighted sections provide the best view of the anal canal, revealing six layers rather than the traditional anatomical description of five layers. From external to internal, these layers are distinguished according to their gray scale: (1) EAS, (2) outer ISS, (3) vertical portion of the levator ani, (4) inner ISS, (5) anal smooth muscle (LRM+IAS), (6) lumen.

Midsagittal anal T1- and T2-weighted sections show the distribution of the anal and perianal structures, including the rectal subserosa, the anal canal, the ISS, the fatty levator fascia, the anorectal junction, the puborectalis, and the EAS.

The T1-weighted axial puborectalis plane shows the structures between the intrahiatal organs and the puborectalis.

2.2.1 Mid-coronal Anal Section

The anal region can be subdivided into an anal portion and a perianal portion (Figs. 2.2, 2.11):

1. The **EAS** appears as the outermost hypointense layer surrounding the lower part of the anal canal. In the coronal plane, the caudal ends of the EAS fold inwards and upwards, forming a double layer. The inner layer is separated from the IAS by the intersphincteric groove (Fig. 2.2).
   The **ISS** is divided into the **outer ISS** and the **inner ISS**. The former is well-appreciated near the anal canal while the latter, as an extension of the perirectal fat, is best seen at a more cranial level. The inner and outer ISSs are spliced by the vertical portion of the levaor ani.
2. The **outer ISS** appears as a layer of high signal intensity. It is delimited by a fatty fascia emerging between the puborectalis and EAS.
3. The **levator ani** is a layer of low signal intensity that is subdivided into vertical and transverse portions. The former inserts into the ISS.
4. The **inner ISS** is a layer of high signal intensity delimited by perirectal fat tissue and the fatty upper levator fascia.

2.2.2 Mid-sagittal Anal Section

The following structures are visible in Fig. 2.12:

- The **anal canal** appears as a tube-like structure consisting of the mucosa, submucosa, and the anal smooth muscle.
- The **subcutaneous sphincter** lies below the caudal end of the imaging anal canal.
- The subcutaneous sphincter and perianal skin create a cover-like structure sealing the imaging anal canal and called the **myocutaneous valve**.
- The **puborectalis** and **deep sphincter** are located behind the anorectal junction.
- The **superficial sphincter** is located anterior and posterior to the anal canal.
- Caudal fibers from the outer layer of the **EAS** extend anteriorly and posteriorly to connect with the bulbocavernosus and the anococcygeal body.
- The plane of the lower pubic symphysis is the **axial puborectalis plane**. It includes the urethra, lower rectum, upper anal canal, and, in men, the prostate.
- The **upper and lower margins of the puborectalis** include the inner and outer ISS and the vertical portion of the levator ani.

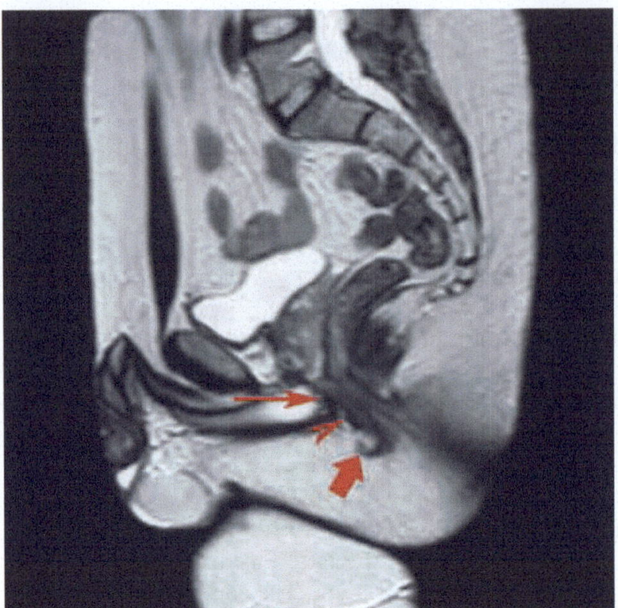

Fig. 2.12 Mid-sagittal anal section. Sagittal T2-weighted image. EAS: subcutaneous (*thick arrow*) and superficial (*arrowhead*) portions; superficial transverse perineal muscle (*thin arrow*)

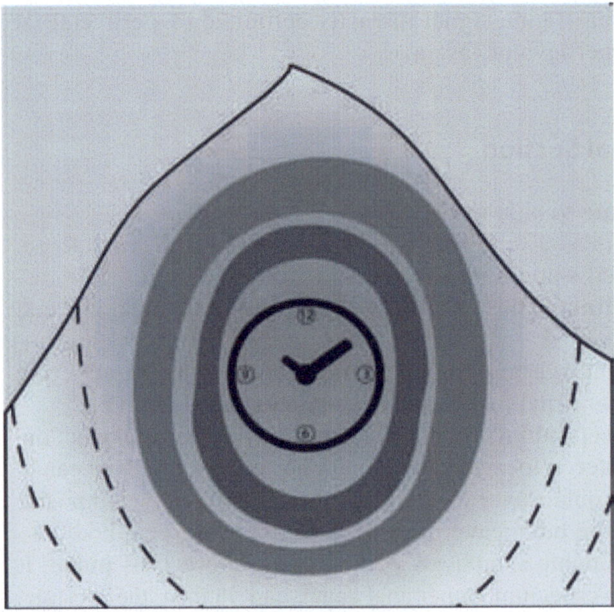

Fig. 2.13 Axial anal section. The "anal clock"

2.2.3 The Anal Clock

Surgeons describe the site and direction of fistulous tracts by referring to the "anal clock", which is the view of the anal region from the feet of the patient, who lies in a lithotomy position. This view is exactly the same as the MRI view in axial planes (Fig. 2.13). Thus, the anterior perineum is located at the 12 o'clock position and the natal cleft at the 6 o'clock position. The left and right lateral aspects of the anal canal are located at the 3 o'clock and 9 o'clock positions, respectively.

References

1. Barleben A, Mills S (2010) Anorectal anatomy and physiology. Surg Clin N Am 90:1-15
2. Guo M, Gao C, Li Det al (2010) Pelvic floor images: anatomy of the levator ani muscle. Dis Colon Rectum 53:1542-1548
3. Hussain SM, Stoker J, Schouten WR et al (1996) Fistula in ano: endoanal sonography versus endoanal MR imaging in classification. Radiology 200:475-481
4. Li D, Guo M (2007) Morphology of the levator ani muscle. Dis Colon Rectum 11:1831-9
5. Kinugasa Y, Arakawa T, Abe TS, et al (2011) Anatomical reevaluation of the anococcygeal ligament and its surgical relevance. Dis Colon Rectum 54:232-237
6. Morren GL, Beets-Tan RG, Van Engelshoven JMA (2001)Anatomy of the anal canal and perineal structures as defined by phased-array magnetic resonance imaging. Br J Surg 88:1506-1512
7. Netter D (1962) Lower digestive tract. In: Digestive System. Elsevier, Teterboro
8. Rociu E, Stoker J, Eijkemans MJC et al (2000) Normal anal sphincter anatomy and age- and sex-related variations at high-spatial-resolution endoanal MR imaging. Radiology 217:395-401
9. Singh K, Reid WMN, Berger LA (2002) Magnetic resonance imaging of normal levator ani anatomy and function. Obstet Gynecol 99:433-438
10. Standring S (2008) Perineum. The anatomical basis of clinical practice. In: Gray's anatomy, vol. 2, 40th edition. Elsevier, Philadelphia
11. Stoker J (2009) Anorectal and pelvic floor anatomy. Best Pract Res Clin Gastroenterol 23:463-475
12. Szurowska E, Wypych J, Elzycka-Swieszewska (2007) Perianal fistulas in Crohn's disease: MRI diagnosis and surgical planning. Abdom Imaging 32:705-718
13. Villa C, Pompili G, Franceschelli G et al (2011) Role of magnetic resonance imaging in evaluation of the activity of perianal Crohn's disease. Eur J Radiol Feb 10. [Epub ahead of print]

Ultrasound Anatomy of the Anorectal Region

3

Giovanni Maconi, Elisa Radice and Giulio A. Santoro

3.1 Introduction

Imaging of the rectum, anorectal junction, and surrounding tissues has always been challenging, including technically, especially when conventional radiological techniques such as computed tomography (CT) and barium studies are used. However, during the past few decades, magnetic resonance imaging (MRI) and sonography have significantly improved visualization of the anorectum and of perianal diseases.

Sonographic assessment of the anal canal and distal rectum is now routinely obtained using endocavitary probes, which combine high spatial resolution with real-time and relatively simple technical evaluation, further improved by recent three-dimensional assessment capabilities [1]. However, the anorectal and perianal regions also can be examined in a transperianeal approach, which combines the advantages of transanal sonography with low cost, wide availability, and non-invasiveness, resulting in an attractive alternative procedure, especially in pregnant woman and in children.

3.2 Anatomy of the Anal Canal

The anal canal is the most distal portion of the gastrointestinal tract, beginning at the anorectal line and ending at the anal verge. It is 3–4 cm in length and its lumen is divided into three parts: the colorectal zone, with columnar mucosa identical to the distal rectal mucosa; the transitional zone, which contains sev-

G. Maconi (✉)
Gastroenterology Unit, Department of Biomedical and Clinical Sciences
Luigi Sacco University Hospital
Milan, Italy
e-mail: giovanni.maconi@unimi.it

M.Tonolini and G. Maconi (eds.), *Imaging of Perianal Inflammatory Diseases*,
DOI: 10.1007/978-88-470-2847-0_3, © Springer-Verlag Italia 2013

eral epithelial variants; and the cutaneous zone, with squamous epithelium [2]. The dentate line, namely, the mucocutaneous junction at the transitional zone, is the site of the largest number of anal glands. These may be implicated in the development of perianal sepsis.

The anal sphincter is composed of an involuntary smooth-muscle inner component, the internal anal sphincter, continuous proximally with the circular muscle fibers of the muscularis propria of the rectum, and the voluntary striated muscle of the external anal sphincter. The internal anal sphincter is discontinuous in the outer third of the anal canal whereas the external sphincter forms a sling-like band surrounding the canal in continuity with the levator ani and puborectalis muscles.

3.3 Normal Ultrasound Anatomy of the Anal Canal and Sphincter Complex

At transanal ultrasound, the anorectal junction is recognized as a puborectalis sling, which creates a hyperechoic U-shaped structure located around the posterior wall of the anal canal, with the anterior aspect comprising the hypoechoic perineal body (Fig. 3.1). The puborectalis and transverse perineal muscles demarcate the proximal portion of the anal canal. The former blends into the external sphincter in the middle part of the canal, creating a complete ring anteriorly (Fig. 3.1).

The internal anal sphincter forms the innermost muscular layer and is the terminal condensation of the circular rectal smooth muscle. It extends from

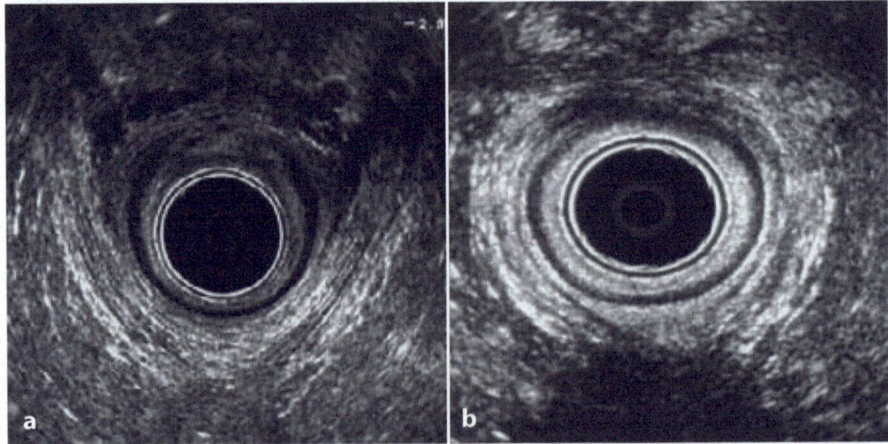

Fig. 3.1 Proximal portion of the anal canal at transanal ultrasound. **a** Anal canal at the level of the anorectal junction as recognized by the puborectalis sling, which creates a hyperechoic U-shaped formation around the posterior wall of the anal canal. **b** Middle portion of the canal. The puboectalis muscle blends with the external sphincter, creating a complete ring

the anorectal junction to 1 cm below the dentate line and is composed of smooth muscle fibers. The internal anal sphincter is seen as a hypoechoic symmetric ring (Fig. 3.2) and is best visualized in the middle part of the anal canal, where it is thickest and uniformly hypoechoic. It is sharply demarcated from the heterogeneous subepithelial tissues medially and the longitudinal muscle laterally.

The circular-shaped external anal sphincter is the outermost muscle of the distal anal canal. While shorter anteriorly in women, it extends approximately 1 cm beyond the internal anal sphincter (Fig. 3.3). The deep part of the external anal sphincter is fused with or intimately related to the puborectalis muscle. Anteriorly, it is closely related to the superficial transverse muscle of the perineum and perineal body, which is seen as a hypoechoic anterior region on transanal ultrasound. The external anal sphincter shows a fibrillar pattern of fine parallel hyperechoic lines in the proximal third of the anal canal (deeper part of the external anal sphincter) which become more homogeneous in the distal third (superficial or subcutaneous part of the external anal sphincter). Although the external sphincter and longitudinal muscle are relatively heterogeneous, they can be distinguished by performing the examination with 10-MHz transducers. Between the two cylindrical layers of the sphincters is the

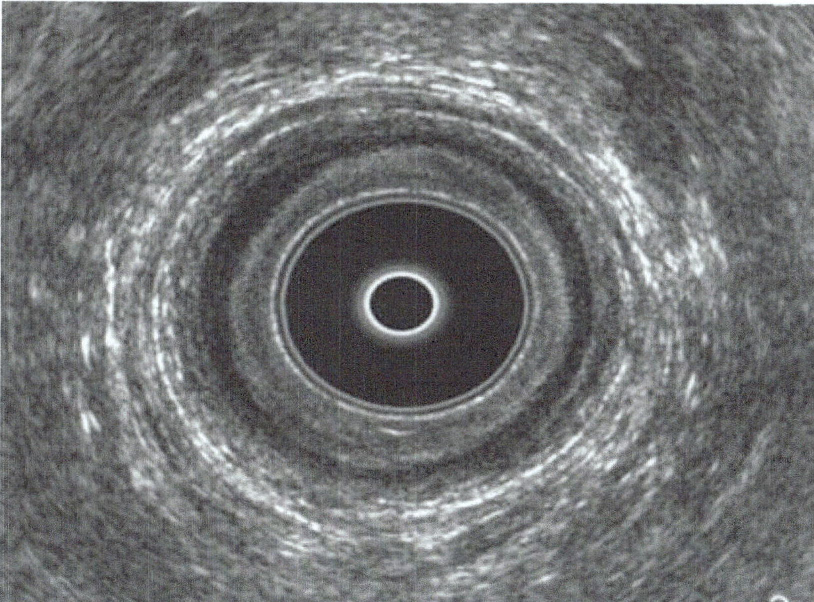

Fig. 3.2 Internal anal sphincter at transanal ultrasound. Tranverse section of the internal anal sphincter, observed as thick hypoechoic symmetric ring in the middle of the anal canal. It is sharply demarcated from heterogeneous subepithelial tissues medially and the longitudinal muscle laterally

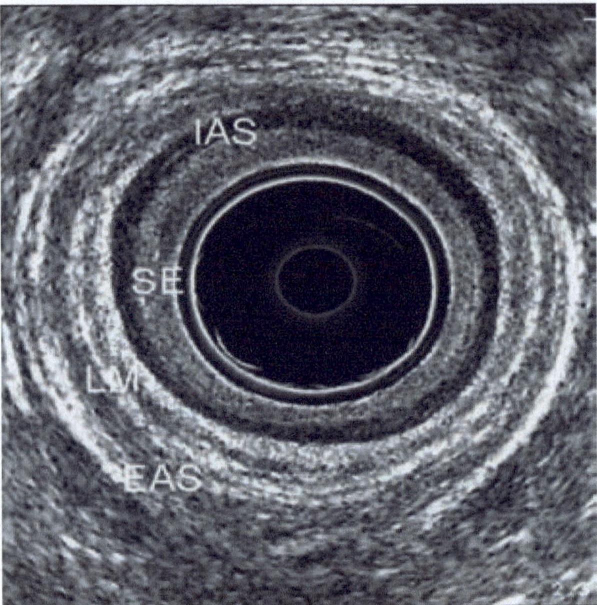

Fig. 3.3 External anal sphincter at transanal ultrasound. Transverse section of the external anal sphincter observed as a circular structure with a typical fibrillar pattern whose deep parts are fused with the puborectalis muscle. *IAS* internal anal sphincter, *SE* subepithelial tissue, *LM* longitudinal muscle, *EAS* external anal sphincter

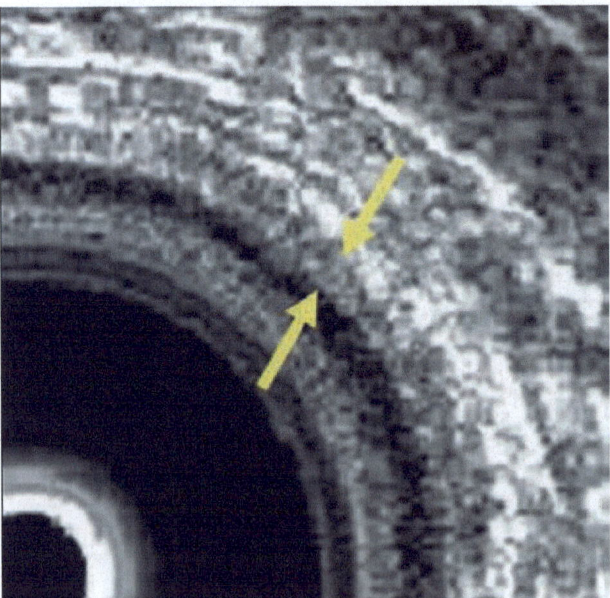

Fig. 3.4 Intersphincteric space at trans-anal ultrasound. It is visible as an hyperechoic band inside the hypoechoic longitudinal muscle (*arrows*)

intersphincteric space, which is visible on transanal sonography as a hyperechoic band sometimes together with a hypoechoic longitudinal muscle, the latter being the continuation of the rectal wall (Fig. 3.4). Therefore, the intersphincteric space may show mixed echogenicity.

Measurements of muscle thickness are clinically important because they are central to the diagnosis of sphincter atrophy and the assessment of fecal incontinence. Transanal ultrasound enables reliable measurement only of internal sphincter thickness, whereas with MRI, especially endoanal MRI, all sphincter components can be reliably measured [3]. Internal sphincter thickness increases with age but is thinner in patients with idiopathic degeneration and abnormally thick in patients with solitary rectal ulcer syndrome [4]. In adults, an internal sphincter thickness measurement that is < 2 mm or > 4 mm is considered abnormal regardless of patient age [4]. However, the external sphincter cannot be measured with confidence presumably because its borders are more difficult to define at transanal sonography. With the use of a high-frequency transducer (10 MHz) greater resolution and precision than were previously achievable can now be obtained [5].

In women, the perineal body separates the anus from the vagina. It is the central portion of the perineum, where the external anal sphincter, the bulbospongious, and the superficial and deep transverse perineal muscles meet. The presence of a thick, contractile perineal body is suggestive of a normal anal sphincter complex [6]. The thickness of the perineal body is defined as the distance between the sonographic reflection of the fingertip placed in the vagina and the inner border of the internal anal sphincter and then the outer border of the subepithelial layer at the level of the mid-anal canal (Fig. 3.5). According to the literature, the normal thickness of the perineal body in women is ≥ 12 mm.

The mucosa and submucosa of the anal canal are seen as a mixed echogenicity gray layer medial to the internal anal sphincter.

As in trans-anal ultrasound, the normal transperineal sonographic appearance of the anal sphincter complex shows: the internal sphincter, a thickened muscle of approximately 3 mm surrounded by the striated external sphincter: this is a slightly thicker structure, measuring approximately 5 mm and with mixed echogenicity (Fig. 3.6). However, images obtained with transperineal sonography may vary according to the different cross-sections. Transverse cross-sections show the same concentric layers obtained by conventional transanal sonography.

3.4 Normal Ultrasound Anatomy of the Rectal Wall and Mesorectum

Optimal imaging of the rectal wall reveals a five-layer structure. The inner white line represents the interface of the mucosal surface of the rectal wall with the contents of the rectum. The inner black line represents the mucosa and

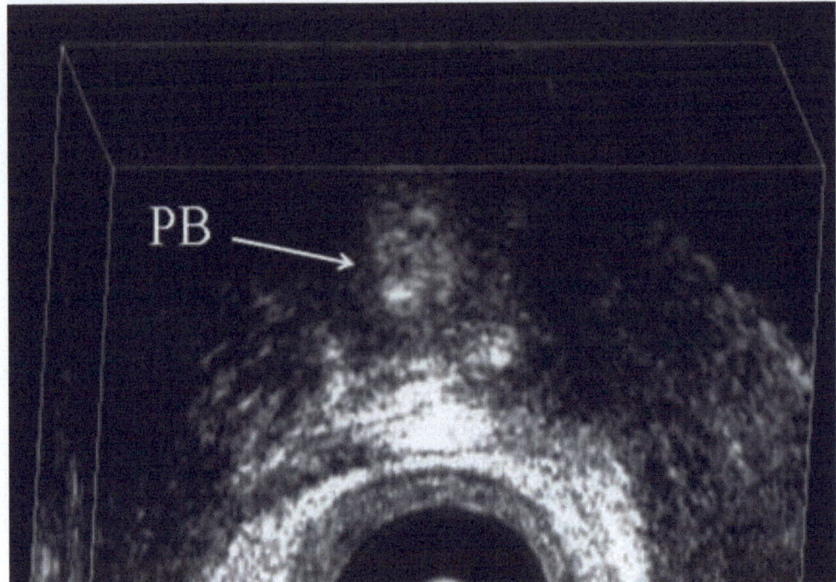

Fig. 3.5 Perineal body (*PB*) at transanal ultrasound. In women, the perineal body separates the anus from the vagina. It can be identified as the distance between the sonographic reflection of the fingertip when placed in the vagina and the inner border of the internal anal sphincter and then the outer border of the subepithelial layer at the level of the mid-anal canal

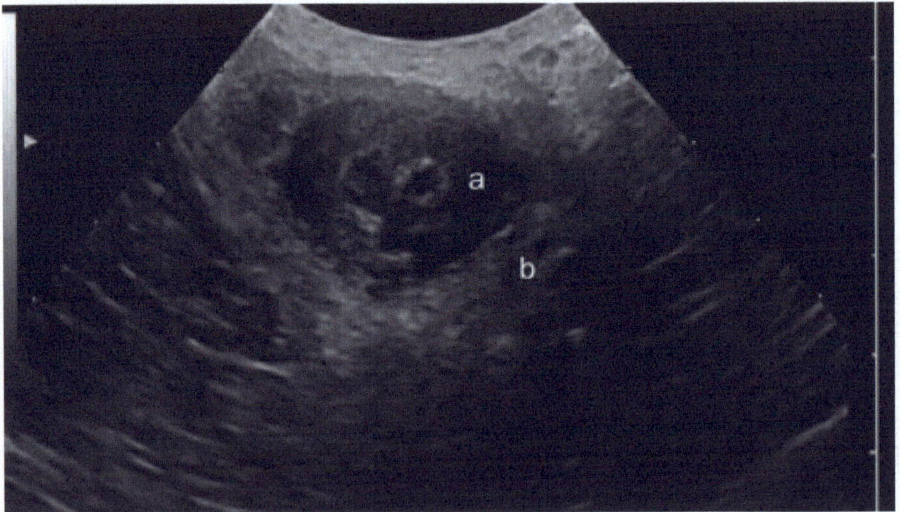

Fig. 3.6 Anal sphincter complex at transperineal ultrasound. Transverse, translabial, cross-section appearance of the anal sphincter complex, showing the internal (*a*) and external (*b*) anal sphincters

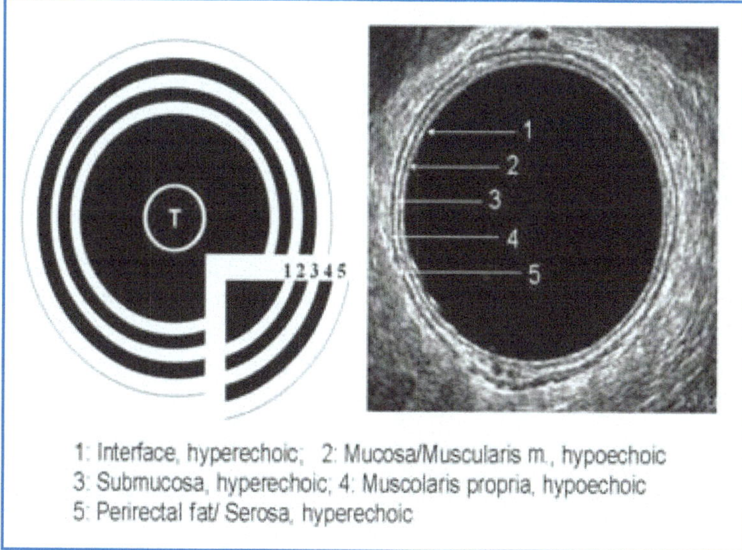

Fig. 3.7 Trans-rectal ultrasound appearance of normal rectal wall. *1* Interface of the balloon and the mucosal surface of the rectal wall; *2* mucosa and muscularis mucosa; *3* submucosa; *4* muscularis propria; *5* interface of the muscularis propria and perirectal fat

muscularis mucosa, and the middle white line indicates the submucosa. The outer black line represents the muscularis propria and the outer white line corresponds to the interface of the muscularis propria and the perirectal fat (Fig. 3.7). Clear distinction of these layers is mandatory especially in the staging of rectal cancer, because infiltration of the rectal wall can differ significantly. It is also important to image the mesorectum and surrounding tissues in order to determine the presence of lymph nodes. Usually, normal lymph nodes are not detected with ultrasound. However, in patients with rectal tumors or anorectal inflammatory conditions, any hypoechoic structures in the surrounding tissues are suspicious for lymph nodes. Metastatic lymph nodes are usually round and hypoechoic, while inflammatory lymph nodes are more often oval and irregular in shape. They must be distinguished from blood vessels running through the mesorectum, which branch and elongate in longitudinal fashion such that they seem to extend further than would be expected based on their diameter.

References

1. Berton F, Gola G, Wilson SR (2007) Sonography of benign conditions of the anal canal: an update. Am J Roentgenol 189:765-73
2. Godlewski G, Prudhomme M (2000) Embryology and anatomy of the anorectum: basis of surgery. Surg Clin North Am 80:319-43

3. Beets-Tan RGH, Morren GL, Beets GL, et al (2001) Measurement of anal sphincter muscles: endoanal US, endoanal MR imaging, or phased array MR imaging? A study with healthy vsolunteers. Radiology; 220:81-9
4. Stoker J, Halligan S, Bartram C (2001) Pelvic floor imaging: state of the art. Radiology 218:621-41
5. Frudinger A, Halligan S, Bartram CI et al (2002) Female anal sphincter: age related differences in asymptomatic volunteers with high frequency endoanal US. Radiology 224:417-23
6. Zetterström JP, Mellgren A, Madoff RD, et al (1998) Perineal body measurement improves evaluation of anterior sphincter lesions during endoanal ultrasonography. Dis Colon Rectum 41:705-13
7. Rubens DJ, Strang JG, Bogineni-Misra S et al (1998) Transperineal sonography of the rectum: anatomy and pathology revealed by sonography compared with CT and MR imaging. AJR Am J Roentgenol 170: 637-42

Section II

Perianal Inflammatory Diseases

Crohn's Disease

4

Andrea Cassinotti

4.1 Disease Spectrum

Inflammatory bowel diseases (IBD), which include Crohn's disease (CD) and ulcerative colitis (UC), are chronic inflammatory diseases of the gastrointestinal tract [1]. IBD cause significant gastrointestinal symptoms, among which are diarrhea, abdominal pain, bleeding, anemia, and weight loss. They are also associated with a spectrum of extraintestinal manifestations, such as arthritis, ankylosing spondylitis, sclerosing cholangitis, uveitis, iritis, pyoderma gangrenosum, and erythema nodosum.

The inflammatory process in CD can involve any part of the digestive tract, from the mouth to the anus, although the distal ileum and/or the colon are the most frequent localizations. Given its typical transmural inflammation, CD can be associated with intestinal complications, particularly strictures, fistulae, and abscesses. Therefore, according to its clinical behavior, CD can be categorized as *luminal* (or *inflammatory*), *fistulizing-penetrating* (with the development of internal/external fistulae, abscess, perforation), or *stricturing* (with the development of intestinal stenosis, posing the risk of bowel obstruction). The phenotype of CD changes with longer follow-up periods: during the first few years, inflammatory forms predominate whereas after 40 years most patients have experienced complications and are classified as having penetrating or stricturing disease [2].

Perianal lesions are a common feature of CD and include anal skin tags, hemorrhoids, anal fissures and ulcers, anorectal strictures, perianal fistulas and abscesses, rectovaginal fistulas, or even carcinoma [3]. In particular, peri-

A. Cassinotti (✉)
Gastroenterology Unit, Luigi Sacco University Hospital
Milan, Italy
e-mail: andreacassinotti@libero.it

M.Tonolini and G. Maconi (eds.), *Imaging of Perianal Inflammatory Diseases*,
DOI: 10.1007/978-88-470-2847-0_4, © Springer-Verlag Italia 2013

anal fistulae are a frequent complication of CD, occurring in around one third of all such patients [4].

Perianal fistulating CD represents a distinct disease phenotype that appears to be separated from luminal fistulating disease, based on differences in disease behavior and therapeutic strategies [5]. The Vienna Classification for CD was devised in 1998 to categorize the diverse CD phenotypes, recognizing the heterogeneity of the disease, but it did not distinguish between perianal and luminal fistulae [6]. Only the recent Montreal modification (2005) provides a separate modifier for perianal disease, which is not necessarily associated with intestinal fistulizing disease, thus underlining the now recognized importance of this phenotype with respect to its impact on disease prognosis and optimal treatment options [7].

4.2 Epidemiology and Natural History

Crohn's disease generally begins in young adulthood and lasts throughout the affected individual's lifetime. For reasons that have yet to be determined, its incidence is increasing worldwide. Unfortunately, the disease is incurable and exerts a significant impact on the quality of life, capacity for work, disability, and health care resources.

Most data on the epidemiology and natural history of IBD have been taken from population-based studies performed in Scandinavia and in Olmsted County, Minnesota, during the years 1950–1970. Disease progression and prognosis has greatly changed with the introduction of corticosteroids in the 1950s, immunosuppressants in the 1970s, and, more recently, biologics. Although these treatments do not have severe complications and improve the quality of life, it is not clear whether they are able to modify the long-term course of the disease.

The highest incidences of CD are reported in northern Europe, the United Kingdom, and North America. There is a high prevalence of IBD among Jewish populations. The peak age for CD occurrence is 20–30 years. Some studies have reported a second peak at 60–70 years, but this has yet to be confirmed. Both genders are involved and smokers have both a higher risk of CD and a worse prognosis.

In the literature, the incidence of perianal inflammation in patients with CD ranges from 25% to 80% [8]. In a community-based study there was a 50% cumulative risk of developing a fistula, including perianal fistula in 26% at 20 years [9]. In approximately 10% of patients with CD, perianal fistula is the initial manifestation, usually preceding the diagnosis by several years; less than 5% of patients have perianal disease as a unique disease manifestation [10].

There are several factors that influence the development of perianal disease, including gender, age, and disease location. Some studies report an increased incidence of perianal fistulae in males, whereas this has not been confirmed in other patient cohorts. Age at disease onset appears to influence the development of perianal lesions, with younger patients at greatest risk. Moreover, fistulae are most common when colonic disease, in particular distal colonic disease, is present. For example, patients with Crohn's colitis were more than three times as likely to develop perianal fistulae as those with ileitis.

Perianal lesions characterize a more aggressive CD phenotype, especially if they are present at the initial diagnosis [11]. Penetrating complications requiring surgical drainage, with a risk of incontinence, are common in these patients. Moreover, patients who undergo surgery for an abscess, fistula, or peritonitis have an increased risk for developing further penetrating complications.

4.3 Pathogenesis

Crohn's disease is a multifactorial disorder of unknown etiology. The pathogenesis likely involves genetic, environmental, and immunological factors. A current theory of IBD development is based on a disregulated immune response, leading to intestinal disease by an altered innate and adaptive immunity in which there is unlimited activation of the immunological mechanisms of inflammation [12].

In CD, antigen-presenting cells and macrophages produce mainly interleukin-12 (IL-12) and IL-18, resulting in a Th1-type polarization and the production of pro-inflammatory cytokines, including tumor necrosis factor-α (TNF-α), interferon-α (IFN-α), and IL-2. Subsequently, these cytokines stimulate antigen-presenting cells to secrete other cytokines, including IL-1, IL-6, IL-8, IL-12, and IL-18, thus leading to a self-sustained cycle. Additionally, other molecules involved in leukocyte trafficking (adhesion molecules), chemokines, and tissue repair molecules are likewise crucial in the pathogenesis of CD.

The pathogenesis of perianal fistulas, despite the prevalence of fistulas in CD, is poorly understood. There are two theories: the first suggests that fistulas begin as deep penetrating ulcers, and the second that fistulas result from anal gland abscesses [13]. Overall, however, it is believed that, as with luminal CD, the etiology of perianal CD involves microbiological, genetic (susceptibility locus on chromosome 5), and immunological factors [14]. This could explain the aggressive and chronic behavior of perianal lesions.

4.4 Medical Therapy: Conventional and New Therapies

In CD, the choice of treatment depends on disease activity and extent as well as patient acceptance. The main therapeutic goals are related to the improvement of the patient's quality of life by inducing and maintaining remission, preventing and treating complications, restoring nutritional deficits, providing appropriate psychosocial support, and modifying the course in those with aggressive disease.

Treatment of perianal CD includes medical and/or surgical options. The primary aim is to heal the perianal lesions but in many cases, because of the aggressiveness of the disease, the physician's role is to relieve symptoms and treat complications. The percentage of spontaneous healing for perianal fistulas is very low, ranging from 6% to 13% in the placebo arm of two controlled studies [15, 16].

Drugs with definite or potential efficacy for treating perianal CD include antibiotics (metronidazole and ciprofloxacin), immunosuppressants (azathioprine and 6-mercaptopurine), calcineurin inhibitors (cyclosporine and tacrolimus), and biologic agents (infliximab, adalimumab, and certolizumab) [17].

In the ECCO consensus statement, antibiotics and azathioprine or 6-mercaptopurine are considered the first-line therapy in complex perianal disease, and infliximab or adalimumab is reserved as second-line treatment in case of failure [18]. In the AGA technical review, infliximab is recommended for the treatment of complex perianal disease along with azathioprine or 6-mercaptopurine and antibiotics for the induction phase. Maintenance is recommended with azathioprine or 6-mercaptopurine, in some cases in association with infliximab [3]. More recently, in the Italian guidelines, anti-TNF-α agents were considered the first-line therapy for perianal disease [19].

4.4.1 Antibiotics

Antibiotics are used as first-line treatment for fistula healing, as well as for abscesses and infection associated with fistulas. Despite the widespread use of antibiotics for the treatment of perianal CD, there is a lack of controlled studies in the literature and the data have mostly been derived from small sample size trials. In these studies, the clinical response generally occurred after 6–8 weeks, as decreased drainage, while fistula closure was uncommon and symptoms tended to recur after the end of treatment. In a recent randomized comparison, only four of ten patients responded to ciprofloxacin compared to one of eight on metronidazole and one of seven on placebo [20]; the study was based on a small sample size and these differences were not significant.

Antibiotics are also used as a bridge to immunosuppressive therapy with azathioprine [21] or as an adjuvant to biological therapy with infliximab [22].

4.4.2 Immunosuppressants

Azathioprine (AZA) and 6-mercaptopurine (6-MP) are immunosuppressive agents effective in inflammatory and post-operative CD; in the treatment of perianal disease, they have only been assessed in retrospective studies. A recent meta-analysis of three studies failed to show a significant superiority of AZA/6MP over placebo in fistulizing disease, finding a clinical response of 55% vs. 29%, with an OR of 4.68 (95% CI 0.6–36.7) [23].

Several uncontrolled case series reported the use of intravenous cyclosporine in patients with perianal CD resistant to traditional therapy, but the initial response was rapidly lost on drug withdrawal. The effects of tacrolimus, which has a similar mechanism, on fistulizing CD were evaluated in a randomized, double-blind, placebo-controlled, multicenter study: 43% of the tacrolimus-treated patients had fistula improvement compared with only 8% of the placebo group; however fistula remission was comparable in the two groups [16]. More studies are warranted; for now, the use of cyclosporine and tacrolimus in the treatment of fistulizing CD is not recommended.

Methotrexate is used as a third-line therapeutic agent for CD patients who do not tolerate AZA and 6-MP. Although no prospective studies have investigated its use for the treatment of fistulizing CD, in a retrospective study 44% of patients treated with methotrexate had partial or complete fistula closure after 6 months [24].

Studies evaluating therapies such as sargramostim (a granulocyte-macrophage colony-stimulating factor), mycophenolate mofetil (an antimetabolite), and thalidomide concluded that these could be considered in the treatment of perianal CD but that more studies are needed to confirm the use.

4.4.3 Biologic Therapies

The use of anti-TNF-α agents has changed the approach to CD, especially in patients with severe and refractory disease, as TNF-α is believed to play a key role in the pathogenesis of IBD.

Infliximab (IFX) is a murine/human chimeric monoclonal antibody directed toward soluble and membrane-bound TNF-α. Two randomized, double-blind, placebo-controlled trials demonstrated the efficacy of IFX in fistulizing CD [15,25]. Both showed that an induction regimen of three infusions (at weeks 0, 2, and 6) of IFX 5 mg/kg followed by maintenance infusions every 8 weeks can induce and maintain complete perianal fistula closure in significantly more patients than placebo. In some patients, the combination of IFX and seton placement can achieve better results. Adverse events of infliximab include infusion reactions, an increased rate of infections, delayed hypersensitivity reactions, formation of antibodies to infliximab, formation of anti-double-stranded DNA antibodies, and drug-induced lupus.

Adalimumab (ADA) is a fully humanized monoclonal antibody directed toward TNF-α and it has proven effectiveness and efficacy in CD [26]. CD patients, including those with a fistula, should receive an induction dose of adalimumab (160 mg in the USA and 80 mg in Europe), with a second dose (80 mg in the USA and 40 mg in Europe) during week 2; the recommended maintenance dose in both the USA and Europe is 40 mg every other week beginning at week 4 and the dose frequency can be increased to once weekly if there is no response.

The clinical effects of ADA were evaluated in two randomized, double-blind, placebo controlled, short-term (4 weeks) induction trials (the CLASSIC-1 trial and the GAIN study). In both studies, fistula closure was not significantly higher in patients treated with ADA than with placebo. There have been no further prospective controlled trials in which perianal fistula closure was the primary end-point. However, in the CHARM study, ADA was associated with a higher rate of fistula closure than achieved with placebo (30% vs. 13%). Moreover, in the CHOICE trial, ADA effectively maintained fistula healing, even among fistulae no longer responsive to IFX).

Two randomized, double-blind, placebo-controlled trials that investigated the efficacy of certolizumab on fistula closure, for comparison with IFX and ADA, were not sufficiently powered [27, 28]. Thus, the effects of this drug require further study.

Notably, Ng et al. [29] used MRI to evaluate CD perianal fistula closure after anti-TNF-α. Even though the fistulas appeared clinically healed, MRI demonstrated persistence of the fistulous tracts, as also demonstrated by previous studies. Thus, MRI confirmed fistula resolution could be useful to determine the duration of anti-TNF-α therapy.

4.4.5 Other Treatments

A recent Japanese study investigated the effects of adsorptive carbon in patients with fistulizing CD [30]. Improvement was achieved in 37% of patients treated with an oral adsorptive carbon agent (AST-120) compared to 10% of the placebo group; the former group also had a significantly higher rate of remission (29.6% vs. 6.7%). Adsorptive carbon probably reverses abnormalities in the luminal environment and gut microflora.

In an uncontrolled study in patients with perianal CD, carbon dioxide laser ablation was considered an alternative treatment [31].

The injection of fibrin glue into fistulas is a simple and safe procedure [32]. The first series in which this treatment was tested reported good healing rates (52–60%), but recent trials have not achieved the same success. Fibrin glue variants include human granulocyte colony-stimulating factor and autologous mesenchymal adult stem cells [33-35].

More recently, bioprosthetic plugs, incorporating porcine intestinal submucosa, have been used in the treatment of patients with anal fistulas, but in a retrospective review their use was associated with a lower success rate (15%) than previously reported.

Finally, other local therapies currently are under development, including the direct injection into the fistula of tacrolimus, infliximab, and adalimumab; the rationale of this approach is to avoid systemic toxicity.

References

1. Baumgart DC, Sandborn WJ (2007) Inflammatory bowel disease: clinical aspects and established and evolving therapies. Lancet 369:1641-1657
2. Louis E, Collard A, Oger AF et al (2001) Behaviour of Crohn's disease according to the Vienna classification: changing pattern over the course of the disease. Gut 49:777-782
3. Sandborn WJ, Fazio VW, Feagan BG et al (2003) AGA technical review on perianal Crohn's disease. Gastroenterology 125:1508-1530
4. Ardizzone S, Porro GB (2007) Perianal Crohn's disease: overview. Dig Liver Dis 39:957-958
5. Tang LY, Rawsthorne P, Bernstein CN (2006) Are perineal and luminal fistulas associated in Crohn's disease? A population-based study. Clin Gastroenterol Hepatol 4:1130-1134
6. Gasche C, Scholmerich J, Brynskov J et al (2000) A simple classification of Crohn's disease: report of the Working Party for the World Congresses of Gastroenterology, Vienna 1998. Inflamm Bowel Dis 6:8-15
7. Satsangi J, Silverberg MS, Vermeire S et al (2006). The Montreal classification of inflammatory bowel disease: controversies, consensus, and implications. Gut 55:749-753
8. Vermeire S, Van Assche G, Rutgeerts P (2007) Perianal Crohn's disease: classification and clinical evaluation. Dig Liver Dis 39: 959-962
9. Schwartz DA, Loftus EV Jr, Tremaine WJ et al (2002). The natural history of fistulizing Crohn's disease in Olmsted County, Minnesota. Gastroenterology 122:875-880
10. Ingle SB, Loftus EV Jr (2007). The natural history of perianal Crohn's disease. Dig Liver Dis 39:963-969
11. Beaugerie L, Seksik P, Nion-Larmurier I et al (2006) Predictors of Crohn's disease. Gastroenterology 130:650-656
12. Schirbel A, Fiocchi C (2010) Inflammatory bowel disease: established and evolving considerations on its etiopathogenesis and therapy. J Dig Dis 11:266-276
13. Schwartz DA, Pemberton JH, Sandborn WJ (2001) Diagnosis and treatment of perianal fistulas in Crohn disease. Ann Intern Med 135:906-918
14. Tozer PJ, Whelan K, Phillips RK et al (2009) Etiology of perianal Crohn's disease: role of genetic, microbiological, and immunological factors. Inflamm Bowel Dis 15:1591-1598
15. Present DH, Rutgeerts P, Targan S et al (1999) Infliximab for the treatment of fistulas in patients with Crohn's disease. N Engl J Med 340:1398-1405
16. Sandborn WJ, Present DH, Isaacs KL et al (2003) Tacrolimus for the treatment of fistulas in patients with Crohn's disease: a randomized, placebocontrolled trial. Gastroenterology 125:380-388
17. Ruffolo C, Citton M, Scarpa M et al (2010) Perianal Crohn's disease: is there something new? World J Gastroenterol 17:1939-46
18. Van Assche G, Dignass A, Reinisch W et al (2010) The second European evidence-based Consensus on the diagnosis and management of Crohn's disease: special situations. J Crohns Colitis 4:63-101
19. Orlando A, Armuzzi A, Papi C et al (2011) The Italian Society of Gastroenterology (SIGE) and the Italian Group for the study of Inflammatory Bowel Disease (IG-IBD) Clinical Practice Guidelines: the use of tumor necrosis factor-alpha antagonist therapy in inflammatory bowel disease. Dig Liver Dis 43:1-20
20. Thia KT, Mahadevan U, Feagan BG et al (2009) Ciprofloxacin or metronidazole for the treatment of perianal fistulas in patients with Crohn's disease: a randomized, double-blind, placebo-controlled pilot study. Inflamm Bowel Dis 15:17-24
21. Dejaco C, Harrer M, Waldhoer T et al (2003) Antibiotics and azathioprine for the treatment of perianal fistulas in Crohn's disease. Aliment Pharmacol Ther 18:1113-1120
22. West RL, van der Woude CJ, Hansen BE et al (2004) Clinical and endosonographic effect of ciprofloxacin on the treatment of perianal fistulae in Crohn's disease with infliximab: a double blind placebo-controlled study. Aliment Pharmacol Ther 20:1329-1336

23. Prefontaine E, MacDonald JK, Sutherland LR (2010) Azathioprine or 6-mercaptopurine for induction of remission in Crohn's disease. Cochrane Database of Systematic Reviews 6:CD000545
24. Soon SY, Ansari A, Yaneza M et al (2004) Experience with the use of low-dose methotrexate for inflammatory bowel disease. Eur J Gastroenterol Hepatol 16:921-926
25. Sands BE, Anderson FH, Bernstein CN et al (2004) Infliximab maintenance therapy for fistulizing Crohn's disease. N Engl J Med 350:876-885
26. Hanauer SB, Sandborn WJ, Rutgeerts P et al (2006) Human anti-tumor necrosis factor monoclonal antibody (adalimumab) in Crohn's disease: the CLASSIC-I trial. Gastroenterology 130: 323-333
27. Sandborn WJ, Feagan BG, Stoinov S et al (2007) Certolizumab pegol for the treatment of Crohn's disease. N Engl J Med 357:228-238
28. Schreiber S, Khaliq-Kareemi M, Lawrance IC et al (2007) Maintenance therapy with certolizumab pegol for Crohn's disease. N Engl J Med 357:239-250
29. Ng SC, Plamondon S, Gupta A et al (2009) Prospective evaluation of anti-tumor necrosis factor therapy guided by magnetic resonance imaging for Crohn's perineal fistulas. Am J Gastroenterol 104:2973-2986
30. Fukuda Y, Fujii H, Koganei K et al (2008) Oral spherical adsorptive carbon for the treatment of intractable anal fistulas in Crohn's disease: a multicenter, randomized, double-blind, placebo-controlled trial. Am J Gastroenterol 103:1721-1729
31. Moy J, Bodzin J (2006) Carbon dioxide laser ablation of perianal fistulas in patients with Crohn's disease: experience with 27 patients. Am J Surg 191:424-427
32. Hammond TM, Grahn MF, Lunniss PJ (2004) Fibrin glue in the management of anal fistulae. Colorectal Dis 6:308-319
33. Vaughan D, Drumm B (1999) Treatment of fistulas with granulocyte colony-stimulating factor in a patient with Crohn's disease. N Engl J Med 340:239-240
34. Peiro C, Rodríguez-Montes JA (2005) A phase I clinical trial of the treatment of Crohn's fistula by adipose mesenchymal stem cell transplantation. Dis Colon Rectum 48:1416-1423
35. Garcia-Olmo D, Herreros D, Pascual I et al (2009) Expanded adipose-derived stem cells for the treatment of complex perianal fistula: a phase II clinical trial. Dis Colon Rectum 52:79-86

5 Ulcerative Colitis

Giovanni Maconi, Cristina Bezzio and Sandro Ardizzone

5.1 Introduction

Perianal disease is a well-known complication of Crohn's disease (CD). It is usually associated with a poorer prognosis and frequently requires an intensive therapeutic approach. However, patients with ulcerative colitis (UC) may also have perianal problems to the extent that they represent a relevant aspect of the disease, associated with patient discomfort and worsening of his or her health. For instance, hemorrhoidal bleeding may mimic a relapse of UC, causing anxiety and the risk of inappropriate treatment. Perianal disease (PAD), in the form of perianal fistulas and abscesses, may develop and progress up to severe perianal septic conditions if unrecognized, especially in patients taking immunosuppressants. Furthermore, in UC patients who are candidates for ileal-pouch-anal-anastomosis (IPAA), the recognition and treatment of perianal conditions may be a prognostically relevant issue.

5.2 Ulcerative Colitis

Perianal complications develop in a considerable proportion of patients with UC, with a prevalence ranging from 3.7 to 32%. These lesions include hemorrhoids, anal skin tags, anal strictures, fissures, fistulae, and abscesses [5]. However, their exact prevalence is difficult to estimate since most studies have been retrospective ones and were performed before 1970, when colonic CD and indeterminate colitis were not yet recognized or described. Therefore, it is

G. Maconi (✉)
Gastroenterology Unit, Department of Biomedical and Clinical Sciences
Luigi Sacco University Hospital
Milan, Italy
e-mail: giovanni.maconi@unimi.it

M.Tonolini and G. Maconi (eds.), *Imaging of Perianal Inflammatory Diseases*,
DOI: 10.1007/978-88-470-2847-0_5, © Springer-Verlag Italia 2013

possible that the rates of perianal complications reported thus far are rather high and, consequently, misleading [1, 2, 4, 6-9] (Table 5.1).

The prevalence of hemorrhoidal disease in UC patients vs. the general population has not been prospectively examined. However, it is reasonable to expect that in the former the rates of hemorrhoids are higher and that inflammatory bowel disease (IBD) is a risk factor for hemorrhoid onset, because diarrhea is the main symptom of UC and is related to the occurrence of hemorrhoidal disease.

Surprisingly, despite the prevalence and complications of hemorrhoidectomy, the procedure, when performed in the treatment of UC, has yet to be fully investigated. Currently, it seems that surgical management of hemorrhoids in UC is usually safer than in CD. This conclusion is supported by a single retrospective study which showed that only 2.3% (1/42) of patients with UC and 30% (6/20) of those with CD required rectal excision for complications apparently arising from hemorrhoid treatment [10]. However, it should be considered that surgical hemorrhoidectomy carries the risk of anal strictures and perianal sepsis. Therefore, in UC patients with active rectal disease the degree of rectal disease activity must be assessed and surgical treatment postponed; instead favoring medical treatment or rubber band ligation.

The prevalence of anal skin tags, both those often referred to as "elephant ears" (type 1) and those typically arising from a healed anal fissure, ulcer, or hemorrhoids (type 2), was investigated in a recent prospective study by Bonheur et al. [11]. The authors reported that these lesions may be found in 25% of patients with UC but they are significantly more common in patients with CD (75% of cases), in particular those with colitis. However, these

Table 5.1 Reported rates of perianal complications in UC patients

Author and year	Number of patients	Hemorrhoid	Abscess	Perianal fistula	Recto-vaginal fistula	Anal fissure
Bargen 1929 [8]	693		26 (3.7%)			
Jackman 1954 [7]	200		15 (7.5%)*			9 (4.5%)
Bockus et al. 1956 [6]	125		23 (18%)*			
Edwards & Truelove 1964 [2]	624	129 (20.7%)	26 (4.2%)*		11 (3%)§	
de Dombal et al. 1966 [1]	465		28 (6%)	25 (5.4%)	10 (3.6%)§	57 (12.3%)
Richard et al. 1997 [9]	753	25 (3.3%)	13 (1.7%)	7 (0.9%)		12 (2.2%)
Zabana et al. 2011 [4]	758		37 (5%)*			

* Abscess and fistulae are reported together; § prevalence among the women patients

lesions are more likely to have diagnostic significance than a prognostic impact, although this remains to be confirmed.

Anal stricture in UC has been described only as a complication of IPAA and is discussed below.

Perianal abscesses and/or fistulae in UC have been less well investigated than in CD. A few early studies reported a prevalence varying from 1.7% to 18%, with an average of 4.6%, which concurs with the findings reported in a recent study by Zabana et al. [4]. The latter study showed that these lesions occur in 5% of patients with UC, taking into account those with an initial diagnosis of the disease and in the 4% of patients who maintained the diagnosis (despite PAD) after a diagnostic reassessment. PAD develops more frequently in patients with active UC, in particular immunocompromised patients and those with increased requirements of steroid therapy [4, 9]. It was also recently observed that UC complicated by perianal fistulae shows a greater and earlier requirement for steroids, immunomodulators, and biological therapy, mainly due to the PAD itself, compared with UC without PAD (Table 5.2).

Complex PAD carries relevant prognostic implications. It occurs mainly in patients in whom the initial diagnosis of UC will change to CD or indeterminate colitis and it is a significant risk factor for colectomy. Zabana et al. (2011) showed that in more than one-third of patients with UC and complex PAD the initial diagnosis changed, whereas this was not the case in any patient with simple PAD [4]. This study also showed that the prevalence of colectomy in UC patients with perianal fistulae and abscesses was nearly double that of patients without [4].

5.2 Ileo-Pouch-Anal-Anastomosis

The main perianal complications of ileo-pouch-anal-anastomosis (IPAA) in patients with UC are strictures and fistulae. Symptomatic strictures may develop in up to 16% of patients [12-14]. Usually, the anastomotic stricture takes

Table 5.2 Disease course, major-disease related events and therapeutic approach in UC patients with and without perianal fistulae or abscesses (PAD) (modified from [4])

	UC-PAD n=37	UC-non PAD n=74	P
Proximal spread	7 (19)	9 (12)	ns
Steroids reintroduction	31 (84)	47 (64)	0.019
Immunomodulators	25 (68)	27 (36)	0.002
Biological therapy	8 (22)	5 (7)	0.022
Hospitalization	26 (70)	38 (51)	0.057
Colectomy	9 (24)	8 (11)	0.062

6–9 months to develop [15], appearing as web-like after a stapled IPAA or long and narrow after mucosectomy and a hand-sewn anastomosis. Strictures also may develop as a complication of cuff abscesses or of surgical techniques (e.g., following the use of a small circular stapler head, for mesenteric tension and partial anastomotic separation) [12].

Patients with anastomotic strictures usually present with watery stools, urgency of defecation, straining, and a sensation of incomplete evacuation.

Treatment includes dilatation by digital insertion or the insertion of graduated Hegar's dilators (in this case usually under general anesthesia), subsequently maintained for soft and short strictures with daily self-dilatation using an anal dilator. However, long strictures are less likely to yield to simple dilatation and, like refractory strictures, may require surgical treatment; they are associated with a high failure/stoma rate [12].

Pouch-vaginal fistulae and perianal fistulae develop in up to 5.5% of patients who have undergone IPAA and are usually the result of chronic infection or bowel inflammation, likely from a persistent anastomotic leak or from unrevealed CD [12, 13].

It has been shown that a postoperative diagnosis of CD is associated with a preoperative diagnosis of indeterminate colitis and perianal fistula, whilst a delayed diagnosis of CD, even years after surgery, is associated with preoperative colonic stricture (OR = 2.9), perianal fistula (OR = 2.9), and oral ulceration (OR = 3.8) [16].

Other studies have shown that patients with UC who were treated by IPAA and have preoperative clinical signs favoring the diagnosis of CD are at risk for the development of pouch-related fistulae [16, 17]. However, in patients with UC, pouch-related fistulae may develop also as a consequence of full-thickness inflammation of the rectum, as encountered in severe active disease and in fulminating colitis [18]. In turn, fistulizing disease after IPAA is associated with a high failure/stoma rate (approximately 46%), despite treatment with infliximab and/or azathioprine/6-mercaptopurine.

References

1. de Dombal F, Watts J, Watkinson G, Goligher J (1966) Incidence and management of anorectal abscess, fistula, and fissure in patients with ulcerative colitis. Dis Colon Rectum 9:201–16
2. Edwards F, Truelove SC (1964) The course and prognosis of ulcerative colitis. Part III Complications. Gut 32:1–22
3. Fuzy PZ (1961) Surgical management of anorectal complications of chronic ulcerative colitis. South Med J 54:795–817
4. Zabana Y, Van Domselaar M, Garcia-Planella E et al (2011) Perianal disease in patients with ulcerative colitis: A case-control study. J Crohn's Colitis 5:338-341
5. Hamzaoglu I, Hodin R (2005) Perianal problems in patients with ulcerative colitis. Inflamm Bowel Dis 11:856–9
6. Bockus H, Roth J, Buchman E et al. (1956) Life history of non-specific ulcerative colitis. Relation of prognosis to anatomical and clinical varieties. Gastroenterology 86:549–81

7. Jackman R. (1954) Management of anorectal complications of chronic ulcerative colitis. Arch Intern Med 94:420–4
8. Bargen J (1929) Complications and sequela of chronic ulcerative colitis. Ann Intern Med 3:335–52
9. Richart CS, Cohen Z, Stern HS et al. (1997) Outcome of pelvic pouch procedure in patients with prior perianal disease. Dis Colon Rectum 40:647-652
10. Jeffery PJ, Parks AG, Ritchie JK (1977) Treatment of haemorrhoids in patients with inflammatory bowel disease. Lancet 1:1084-5
11. Bonheur J, Braunstein J, Korelitz BI, Panagopoulos G (2008) Anal skin tags in inflammatory bowel disease: new observations and a clinical review. Inflamm Bowel Dis 14:1236-1239
12. Sagar PM, Pemberton JH (2012) Intraoperative, postoperative and reoperative problems with ileoanal pouches. Br J Surg 99:454-68
13. Hueting WE, Buskens E, van der Tweel I, Gooszen HG, van Laarhoven CJ (2005). Results and complications after ileal pouch anal anastomosis: a meta-analysis of 43 observational studies comprising 9,317 patients. Dig Surg 22:69-79
14. Lewis WG, Kuzu A, Sagar PM, Holdsworth PJ, Johnston D (1994) Stricture at the pouch–anal anastomosis after restorative proctocolectomy. Dis Colon Rectum 37: 120–125
15. Prudhomme M, Dozois RR, Godlewski G, Mathison S, Fabbro-Peray P. (2003) Anal canal strictures after ileal pouch–anal anastomosis. Dis Colon Rectum 46: 20–23
16. Melton GB, Kiran RP, Fazio VW et al. (2010) Do preoperative factors predict subsequent diagnosis of Crohn's disease after ileal pouch-anal anastomosis for ulcerative or indeterminate colitis? Colorectal Dis 12:1026-32
17. Tekkis PP, Fazio VW, Remzi F, et al (2005) Risk factors associated with ileal pouch-related fistula following restorative proctocolectomy. Br J Surg 92:1270-6
18. Warren BF (2004) Classical pathology of ulcerative colitis and Crohn's colitis. J Clin Gastroenterol 38:S33-S35

Cryptogenetic Fistulas

6

Andrea Bondurri, Piergiorgio Danelli and Matteo Marone

6.1 Introduction

Cryptogenic anal fistulas are a significant problem that has affected and continues to effect a large number of people throughout the world, with devastating consequences in terms of quality of life and sense of well being. A fistula is defined as an abnormal connection between two epithelium-lined organs that are not normally connected. An anal fistula is an abnormal connection between the anorectum and the perineum.

The prevalence of this disease is about 8.6 cases per 100,000 population, with a higher prevalence in males than in females (12.3 vs. 5.6 cases per 100,000 population, respectively). The average age of onset is 38.3 years.

An anal fistula is composed of an internal orifice, a tract, and an external orifice. The external orifice can be easily identified during the acute phase of the disease but is more difficult to detect in the chronic disorder. The position of the internal orifice can be predicted according to that of the external orifice based on Goodsall's Law (Fig. 6.1), which states that when the external opening of a fistula is situated anterior to the transverse plane, the internal orifice tends to be located radially. When the external opening lies posterior to the plane, the orifice is usually located in the posterior midline. It is important to differentiate fistulas from other perianal diseases, such as hidradenitis suppurativa, infected inclusion cyst, pilonidal disease, and, in females, Bartholin gland abscess.

Worldwide, cryptoglandular infection is considered the most likely cause of cryptogenic anal fistula. Most people have between six and eight anal glands, varying in location between the internal anal sphincter and the inter-

A. Bondurri (✉)
General Surgery 1, Luigi Sacco University Hospital
Milan, Italy
e-mail: bondurri.andrea@hsacco.it

M.Tonolini and G. Maconi (eds.), *Imaging of Perianal Inflammatory Diseases*,
DOI: 10.1007/978-88-470-2847-0_6, © Springer-Verlag Italia 2013

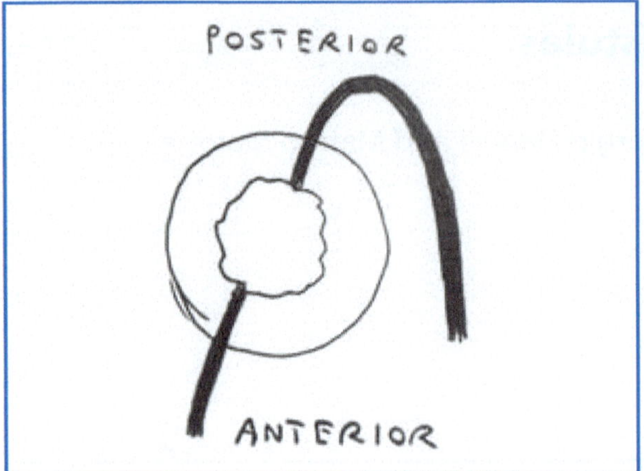

Fig. 6.1 Goodsall's Law

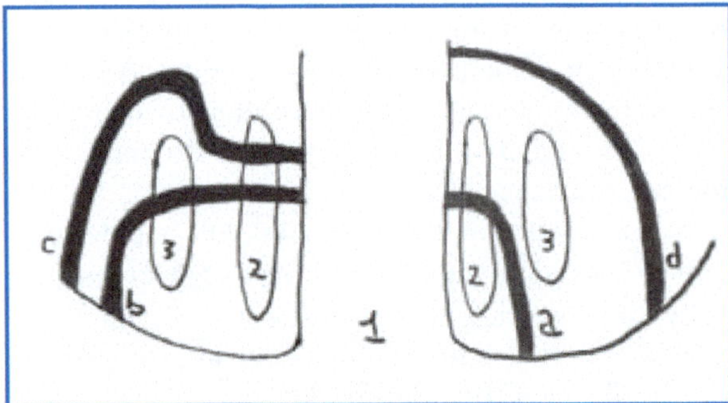

Fig 6.2 The Parks classification. *1* Rectum, *2* internal sphincter, *3* external sphincter, *a* intersphincteric, *b* extrasphincteric, *c* suprasphincteric, *d* transsphincteric

sphincteric groove. The sequence of events leading to fistula formation and its consequences is usually described as obstruction-infection-abscess-fistula. Thus, an obstruction of the gland causes an infection which in turn produces an abscess and then a fistula. However, about 10% of abscesses are due to other causes, such as Crohn's disease, HIV infection, trauma, sexually transmitted diseases, and radiation therapy [1-4].

Fistulas were classified by Parks and colleagues into different types according to their relation to the anal sphincter muscles (Fig. 6.2).

- Intersphincteric fistulas pass through internal sphincter (45% of cases) (Fig. 6.2).
- Transsphincteric fistulas pass through both the internal and external sphincter (30% of cases) (Fig. 6.2).
- Suprasphincteric fistulas pass through the internal sphincter but traverse the external sphincter below the puborectalis muscle (20% of cases) (Fig. 6.2).

- Extrasphincteric fistulas pass the sphincter complex through the ischiorectal fossa to the perianal skin (5% of cases).

This classification is not an abstract one but is genuinely useful as it can predict the risk of fecal incontinence after surgery [5].

Fistulas can also be classified as simple or complex, even if there is no consensus in the literature. Simple fistulas may include submucosal, low transsphincteric, and low intersphincteric fistulas (traversing < 30% of the internal anal sphincter). Complex fistulas tend to be those with multiple external openings, high transsphincteric, suprasphincteric, and extrasphincteric fistulas, high blind extensions, horseshoe tracts, anterior fistulas in female patients, fistulas associated with a high risk of continence disturbance after surgery, and fistulas in Crohn's disease or associated with irradiation.

The great challenges in the treatment of anal fistulas are maintaining continence, achieving rapid healing, the elimination of all septic foci, and reducing the risk of recurrence.

6.2 Surgical Approaches to Fistula Treatment

Medical therapy is not useful for the treatment of anal fistulas even if antibiotic prophylaxis and infliximab may have a therapeutic roles especially in patients with Crohn's disease. Surgical treatment achieves the highest number of fistula closures and is based on several different procedures: fistulotomy, fistulectomy, seton (cutting and non-cutting types), endorectal advancement flaps, fibrin glue, plugs, ligation of fistula tract (LIFT), and video-assisted anal fistula treatment (VAAFT). Before a patient undergoes a surgical procedure, it is important to evaluate the relevance of the problem. This can be performed in two steps: outside the operating theatre, with preoperative examination, and inside the operating theatre, by identifying both orifices of the fistula.

Endosonography is a safe procedure that allows the detection of abnormalities in the anal canal as well as defects of the perianal region, including the fistula tract and abscesses. Moreover, it can identify a fistula as simple or complex. However, it is not always easy to differentiate pathological findings from scars or granulating tracts. Consequently, hydrogen peroxide injection from the external orifice of the fistula, so as to create a gaseous contrast, has been introduced. Another important innovation is 3D axial reconstruction, which generates a multidimensional view of the pathological findings.

MRI is used if initial attempts to determine the internal orifice of the fistula are unsuccessful. It provides better visualization not only of the fistula itself but also of the anatomy of the perineum and of the relationship between the fistula and other organs. Fistulography is a radiological technique that uses X-rays and a water-soluble contrast to demonstrate the fistula tract. Unfortunately, it cannot show the relationship between the fistula and the perineum and is therefore useful only in rare cases. The function of the anal sphincter can be evaluated with anal manometry, which allows the surgeon to choose the best surgical technique [6-8].

6.2.1 Fistulotomy

This is the best procedure for the treatment of single-tract anal fistulas, especially submucosal ones, although some surgeons use this procedure in patients with low intersphincteric or transsphincteric fistulas. Fistulotomy requires the identification of both orifices. This can be performed using a probe and, if needed, hydrogen peroxide injection. The tract is then incised and the granulation tissue removed by curettage. It is important that the excised tissue is sampled in order to allow an histological examination [3, 4, 8].

6.2.2 Fistulectomy

This technique is used in the treatment of transsphincteric fistulas. It is based on the principle that removal of the chronic epithelialized tract will allow healing by secondary intention of healthier tissue. The dissection is carried out from the external orifice while the internal orifice is closed directly. This is a difficult procedure that can result in significant patient morbidity due to the large amounts of tissue and sphincter damage. Success rates are similar to those of fistulotomy, even if subsequent incontinence rates are 15% higher [3, 4, 8].

6.2.3 Seton

The use of a seton has the same purpose as using a wire to cut a block of ice. Thus, a seton is a wire consisting of non-absorbable suture, a drain, or a rubber band. The procedure is recommended for high transsphincteric fistulas, for fistulas involving > 50% of the sphincter, and for anterior fistulas in female patients. There are two main types of setons. Cutting setons cut slowly through the tissue, allowing healing from the inside to the outside in order to reduce the risk of incontinence. Non-cutting setons are used for draining in the acute setting or when other procedures cannot be performed or have failed, in certain inflammatory diseases such as Crohn's disease, or in infectious diseases such as HIV. In the short term, a seton provides rapid and safe relief of the infection without compromising the sphincter complex. It also prevents abscess recurrence and can act as a guide to the internal and external openings for subsequent treatments [3, 4, 8].

6.2.4 Fibrin Glue

Fibrin glue is composed of fibrinogen, thrombin, and calcium and was first used for hemostasis. The glue reacts in about 60 s and promotes the migration of fibroblasts and pluripotent cells, thereby initiating fistula healing. To use the glue, the fistula has to be well cleaned using hydrogen peroxide and curettage, and both orifices have to be closed. Some authors recommend the positioning of a non-cutting seton 6–8 weeks before the procedure [9].

6.2.5 Plugs

These may be biologic (e.g., manufactured from porcine small intestinal mucosa) or non-tissue-derived (e.g., synthetic polymers). The plug is resistant to infection and does not induce a foreign-body reaction. It is inserted into the fistula tract through the internal orifice, trimmed, if needed, and then secured at the internal opening. The latter is important because dislodgement is the primary cause of plug failure. The external opening is left open for drainage in an attempt to reduce the possibility of infection [10].

6.2.6 Ligation of the Intersphincteric Fistula Tract (LIFT)

In this procedure, the fistula tract is identified between the internal and external sphincters and is subsequently divided and tied. The procedure reportedly has a 94% success rate, with no impact on continence. It is considered to be a "sphincter-sparing" technique and is a relatively simple operation. The first step is to identify the intersphincteric groove. Once the skin is incised in this area, a combination of blunt and sharp dissection is used to identify the fistula tract. A modification of the LIFT procedure has recently been described: after the fistula tract is identified and divided, a biologic mesh is placed in the intersphincteric space to act as a barrier [11].

6.2.7 Endorectal Advancement Flaps

The advancement flap is designed to address the pathophysiology of the fistula. The procedure is a sphincter-sparing approach in which the internal opening is closed, in order to remove the source of sepsis, with subsequent healing of the fistula tract by secondary intention. A healthy sleeve of rectal wall is prepared and sutured distal to the internal opening [3, 4, 8].

6.2.8 Video-assisted Anal Fistula Treatment (VAAFT)

A fistuloscope is inserted through the external orifice in order to better identify the internal orifice and all fistula tracts. The internal orifice is closed using a linear stapler, resulting in hermetic closure of the opening. The fistula tract is destroyed using a visually guided electrode [12].

References

1. Shawki S, Wexner SD (2011) Idiopathic fistula-in-ano. World J Gastroenterol 17(28): 3277–3285
2. Whiteford MH (2007) Perianal Abscess/Fistula Disease. Clin Colon Rectal Surg 20(2): 102–109
3. Pescatori M (2011) Ascessi, fistole anali e retto vaginali. Springer, Milan
4. Corman M (2005) Colon & rectal surgery, 5th edn. Lippincot Williams & Wilkins, Philadelphia. pp 7-27, 279-332
5. Parks AG, Gordon PH, Hardcastle JD (1976) A classification of fistula-in-ano. Br J Surg 63:1–12
6. Kim Y, Jin Park Y (2009) Three-dimensional endoanal ultrasonographic assessment of an anal fistula with and without H2O2 enhancement. World J Gastroenterol. 15(38):4810-5
7. El-Tawil AM (2011) Management of fistula-in-ano: an introduction. World J Gastroenterol 17(28): 3271
8. Bleier JIS, Moloo H (2011) Current management of cryptoglandular fistula-in-ano. 17(28): 3286-91
9. Indinnimeo m (2006) Cyanoacrylate glue in the treatment of ano-rectal fistulas. Int J Colorectal Dis 21(8):791-4
10. Ellis CN (2007) Bioprosthetic plugs for complex anal fistulas: an early experience. J Surg Educ 64: 36–40
11. Shanwani A, Nor AM, Amri N (2010) Ligation of the intersphincteric fistula tract (LIFT): a sphincter-saving technique for fistula-in-ano. Dis Colon Rectum 53:39–42
12. Meinero P, Mori L (2011) Video-assisted anal fistula treatment (VAAFT): a novel sphincter-saving procedure for treating complex anal fistulas. Techniques in Coloproctology 15(4):417-22

Sexually Transmitted Diseases

7

Andrea Bondurri, Piergiorgio Danelli and Matteo Marone

7.1 Introduction

Sexually transmitted diseases (STDs) are syndromes caused by bacteria, viruses, fungi, and protozoa that can be acquired and transmitted through sexual activity. In the last two decades, enormous changes have taken place in human sexual activity, resulting in an explosive spread of STDs especially among young people. Today, STDs are the most common types of infections, with about 350 000 000 new cases per year and unparalleled health, social, and economic consequences.

There are at least 25 different STDs, with a range of different symptoms typically involving the genitourinary or anorectal tract. Both may lead to pelvic inflammatory disease or to chronic abscess formation. It is therefore paramount that the surgeon to be knowledgeable about the manifestations, differential diagnosis, and treatment of STDs.

7.2 Human Immunodeficiency Virus

Today, HIV is probably the most important cause of STDs. The most common symptoms are anorectal pain, lumps or warts, rectal bleeding, discharge, and pruritus. Nearly 25% of patients have multiple complaints. Anal condylomata and wide-based anal ulcers are the most frequent lesions observed. The majority of the ulcers are idiopathic, with negative cultures and biopsies. Other lesions include fistulas, abscesses, hemorrhoids, and malignancy [1, 2, 3, 6].

A. Bondurri (✉)
General Surgery 1, Luigi Sacco University Hospital
Milan, Italy
e-mail: bondurri.andrea@hsacco.it

M.Tonolini and G. Maconi (eds.), *Imaging of Perianal Inflammatory Diseases*,
DOI: 10.1007/978-88-470-2847-0_7, © Springer-Verlag Italia 2013

7.3 Proctitis

Proctitis is an inflammation of the rectum restricted to the distal 15 cm of the colon. The causes of sexually transmitted proctitis are gonorrhea (30%), *Chlamydia* (19%), herpes simplex virus type 2 (HSV)-2 (16%), and syphilis (2%). Proctitis is also associated with HIV infection.

Symptoms of proctitis are anorectal pain, tenesmus, constipation, perianal ulcerations, fever, difficulty in urinating, inguinal lymphadenopathy, and diffuse ulcerative, pustular lesions in the distal 5 cm of the rectum.

Neisseria gonorrhoeae, a gram-negative diplococcus, is the main causative agent and infection is more often seen in females. After a bacterial incubation period of 5–7 days, patients report tenesmus, mucopurulent discharge, pruritus and pain [1, 2].

7.4 Herpes

Herpes is caused by herpes simplex virus type 2 (HSV-2) (Fig. 7.1). Symptoms include anal pain, itching, fevers, and myalgias. Red perianal vesicles may be present and their evolution to form ulcers is common. In 50% of patients, lymphadenopathy is present as well [1, 5].

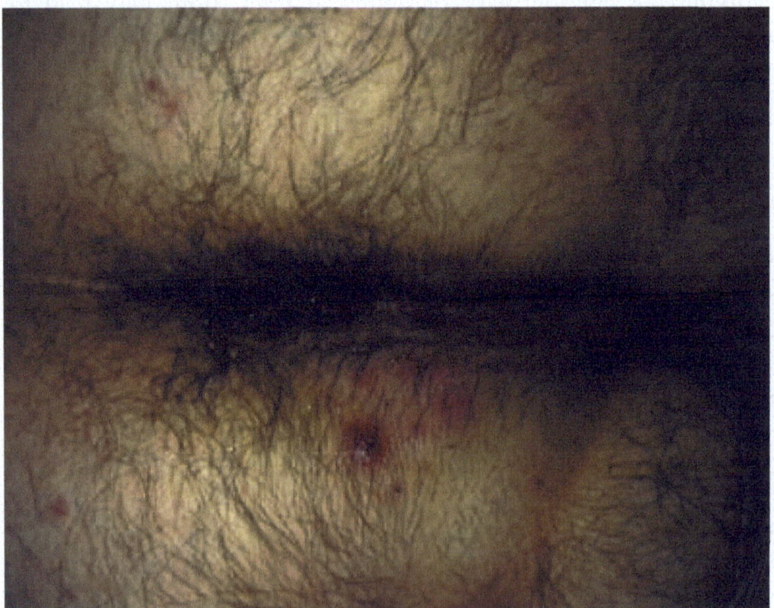

Fig 7.1 HSV proctitis

7.5 Syphilis

Syphilis is caused by the spirochete *Treponema pallidum*. The typical presentation is a single painless anal ulcer (chancre), although other symptoms may be present as well, such as discharge, bleeding, significant pain, and itching.

Secondary syphilis can occur 6–8 weeks after healing of the initial ulcer, especially if the patient was not treated. This stage is characterized by a maculopapular rash, usually located on the palms of the hands and soles of the feet. Genital and anorectal condylomata localize near the initial chancre. There are also systemic symptoms of fever, night sweats, and weight loss [1, 5].

7.6 Lymphogranuloma Venereum

Lymphogranuloma venereum (LGV) is caused by *Chlamydia trachomatis* serotypes L1–L3. Serotype L2 was implicated in a recent outbreak. The symptoms include anal ulceration at the site of inoculation (if present) and painful inguinal lymphadenopathy, also referred to as "buboes". Among patients with LGV, 25% will not develop lymphadenopathy. During a recent outbreak of LGV, most patients had almost exclusively rectal symptoms [2, 5].

7.7 Pox Virus

Molluscum contagiosum is caused by the pox virus. The symptoms include itching and tender pea-sized papules with a plug of white material. However, 50% of patients are asymptomatic.

7.8 Human Papilloma Virus

Condylomata acuminata are warts caused by HPV. These raised pale lesions, occurring externally or internally within the anal canal, can be present singly, in small clusters, or even as large exophytic masses. The symptoms includes friability, itching, and bleeding. Internal warts are usually asymptomatic. Against a background of HIV infection, the warts may be more extensive. An increase in anal cancer among HIV-positive homosexual men with HPV infection has been shown [5, 6].

References

1. Mansour M, Weston LA (2010) Perianal infections: a primer for nonsurgeons. Curr Gastroenterol Rep. 12(4):270-9
2. Hoentjen F, Rubin DT (2012) Infectious proctitis: when to suspect it is not inflammatory bowel disease. Dig Dis Sci 57(2):269-73

3. Shim BS (2011) Current concepts in bacterial sexually transmitted diseases. Korean J Urol 52(9):589-97
4. Aral SO, Blanchard JF (2002) Phase specific approaches to the epidemiology and prevention of sexually transmitted diseases. Sex Transm Infect 78 Suppl 1:i1-2
5. Moroni M, Antinori S, Vullo V (2009) Manuale di malattie infettive. Elsevier, pp. 202-213, 177-194
6. Kasper Dl, Braunwald E, Hauser S et al (2004) Harrison's principles of internal medicine. 16th edn. McGraw-Hill Professional, New York, pp. 1179-1202, 1218-1293

Cancer in Perianal Fistulas

8

Gianluca M. Sampietro, Alice Frontali and Diego Foschi

8.1 Introduction

The presence of a perianal fistula as a complication related to Crohn's disease (CD) was first described by Penner and by Burrill Crohn himself in 1938 [1]. Since then, intense efforts have been made and significant economic resources spent in order to improve the quality of life of patients with inflammatory bowel diseases (IBDs) who also have perianal fistulas. Unfortunately, the results have been poor regardless of the medical or surgical treatment adopted. The incidence of perianal disease is 20–25% in CD patients with terminal ileitis, but it increases to as high as 60% in CD with a colonic location and 92% when the rectum is actively involved [2-4]. In ulcerative colitis (UC) perianal suppurative lesions are less common, but the incidence of perianal abscesses and fistulas is still reported to be between 10% and 15% [5].

The association of colorectal cancer (CRC) and IBD is well established, especially for UC but also for colonic CD (Fig. 8.1). The cumulative incidence in UC patients with pancolitis is reported to be 8.5% and 17.5% at 20 and 30 years of disease duration, respectively [6], while in CD it is 2.9% at 10 years, 5.6% at 20 years, and 8.3% at 30 years, regardless of disease distribution [7]. For those patients with extensive colonic involvement, the cumulative incidence rises to 24% at 30 years [8]. The relative incidence of anal cancer as a proportion of CRC is 14% in CD patients compared to 1.4% in the general population [9]. Malignant transformation of a perianal fistula is rare, but the diagnosis is challenging and treatment is complicated. In the past 30 years, about 200 cases have been reported in the literature, as single case

G.M. Sampietro (✉)
Department of Surgery, Gastroenterology and Oncology, Luigi Sacco University Hospital
Milan, Italy
e-mail: gianluca.sampietro@unimi.it

M.Tonolini and G. Maconi (eds.), *Imaging of Perianal Inflammatory Diseases*,
DOI: 10.1007/978-88-470-2847-0_8, © Springer-Verlag Italia 2013

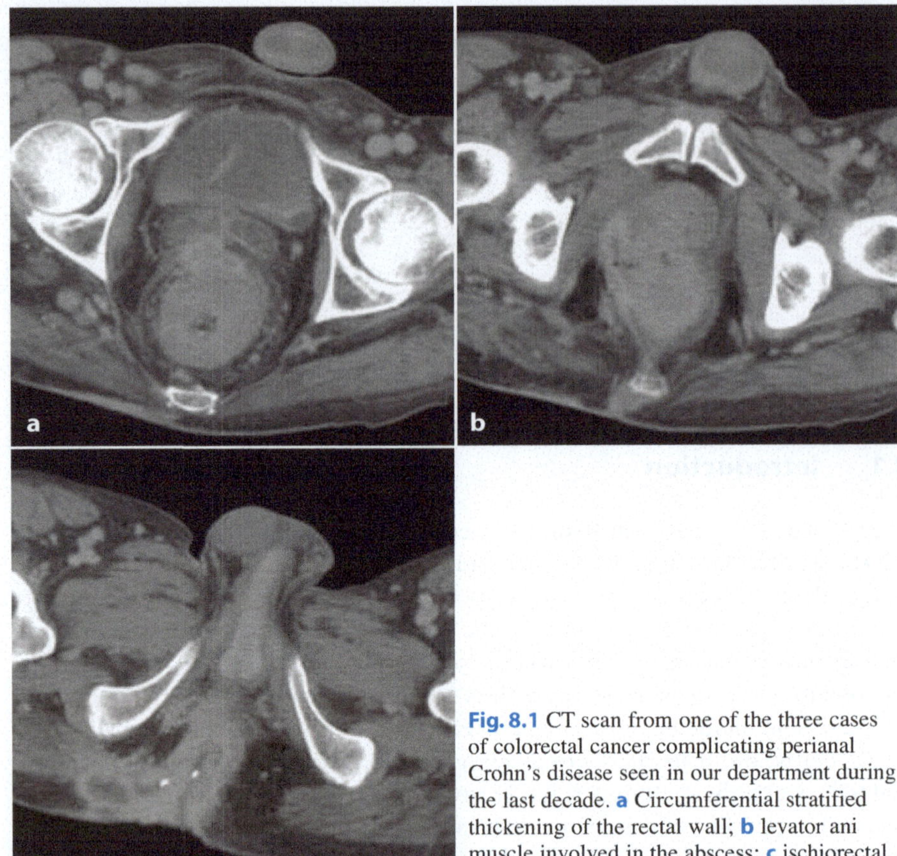

Fig. 8.1 CT scan from one of the three cases of colorectal cancer complicating perianal Crohn's disease seen in our department during the last decade. **a** Circumferential stratified thickening of the rectal wall; **b** levator ani muscle involved in the abscess; **c** ischiorectal abscess and fistula with seton drainage

reports or small series (maximum 8 patients) from referral centers [10-12]. Ky et al. followed more than 1000 patients with complicated perianal CD for 14 years, reporting an incidence of carcinoma related to fistula of 0.7% [10].

8.2 Diagnosis

When malignant transformation of a perianal fistula is suspected, the diagnostic approach is not different from the normal workup for complicated perianal disease as proposed in the Guidelines of the European Crohn's and Colitis Organitazation [13]. Examination under anesthesia (EUA) is considered to be the most sensitive diagnostic tool, with an accuracy of 90% in the hands of an experienced surgeon. It allows concomitant surgery, such as abscess drainage, anal stenosis dilation, and seton placement [14]. Furthermore, a complete set of biopsies can be obtained. Pelvic magnetic resonance imaging (MRI) has an accuracy of 76–100% compared to EUA and may provide additional information [14]. Anorectal ultrasound has an accuracy of 56–100%, especially when performed by experts in conjunction with hydrogen peroxide enhancement [15,16]. The best performance in terms of accuracy is obtained by the combination of EUA with one of the two imaging procedures.

After a diagnosis of CRC is achieved, a complete colonoscopy must be performed in order to assess the presence and extension of mucosal inflammation and to exclude synchronous colonic lesions. According to the guidelines of the National Comprehensive Cancer Network (NCCN version 2.2012), both a total-body computed tomography (CT) scan and measurement of preoperative CEA levels are needed. If the histology is diagnostic of squamous cell carcinoma (SCC), the workup has to be completed with a fine-needle aspiration biopsy of the suspected inguinal lymph nodes, HIV testing, a gynecological exam to exclude cervical cancer, and, in selected cases, positron emission tomography-CT scan. When the patient has extended jejuno-ileal and/or colonic CD, a complete evaluation of the location and behavior of the inflammatory lesions is mandatory due to the critical implications in therapeutic strategy (see 8.3 Treatment). The same preoperative CT scan for cancer staging is in many cases also useful for CD re-staging, providing the appropriate adjustments are made (e.g., entero-CT scan of the abdomen). Unfortunately, detection of cancer at the first visit followed by biopsy confirmation occurs in less than 20% of the cases. Thomas et al., in a recent review of the literature, reported delays in the diagnosis of adenocarcinoma and SCC (non-human-papillomavirus type 16 correlated) of 6.2 and 5.4 months, respectively [17]. Adenocarcinoma is the most common cancer type (60–70%) (Fig. 8.2). At the time of diagnosis, affected women are younger (47 vs. 53 years), have a shorter disease duration (18 vs. 24 years), and a shorter history of perianal disease (8.3 vs. 16 years) than is the case in affected men [17].

8.3 Treatment

Since a cancer complicating perianal disease in IBD is rare, the following indications for treatment are based only on anecdotal case reports and speculative considerations. A cancer originating in a perianal fistula, whether or not it has an intraluminal portion, spreads by definition *outside* the rectal wall, potentially involving soft tissues, muscles, gynecological and urological structures, and even bones. Preoperative staging is difficult to standardize, but according to the different staging systems this kind of cancer is usually classified as T4b or Dukes D, with all the surgical and medical therapeutic implications. In Figures 8.1 and 8.2 are reported the CT scan and EUA findings of a patient with perianal adenocarcinoma extended to the extraluminal pelvic structures. However, in a patient with IBD who is diagnosed with cancer, two major considerations have to be made. On the one hand, these patients are almost always under treatment with immunosuppressive and/or biological therapy in order to con-

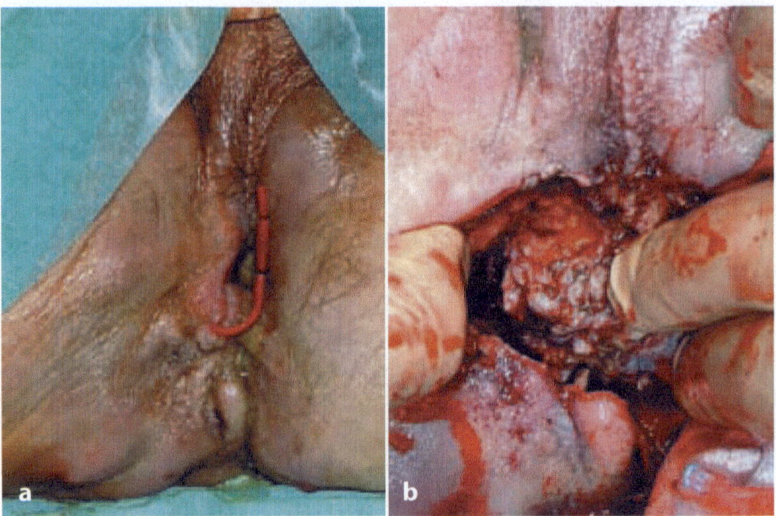

Fig. 8.2 a Clinical presentation of a patient's perineum, showing scars from previous perianal disease, a seton drainage in place, and recurrent fistula and abscess. **b** Adenocarcinoma arising from the perianal fistula invading soft tissues and muscles of the right perineum

trol inflammation. These treatments have to be promptly stopped if ongoing and are absolutely contraindicated in the future. Nonetheless, the problem of maintaining the IBD in remission after surgery for cancer remains unresolved. On the other hand, during treatment with cytotoxic drugs, patients with IBDs will be at high risk of developing complications, such as severe diarrhea, luminal bleeding, enhanced toxic effects, and flare of the inflammation itself [18].

Furthermore, in IBD patients, no data are available regarding specific therapeutic indications for the underlying inflammatory disease during radio- and chemotherapy. Continuous-infusion 5-FU alone, in combination with either leucovorin or oxaliplatin (FOLFOX), seems to be tolerated best, while bolus infusions of 5-FU and combination therapy of irinotecan with 5-FU should be avoided because of severe diarrhea and the possibility of sepsis. Although it is theoretically possible that cetuximab could adversely alter IBD activity, clinical experience in CRC patients has not shown any significant gastrointestinal side effects. Bevacizumab, however, has been associated with rare episodes of intestinal perforation and should thus be used with extreme caution in patients who have IBD [18]. Of course, different scenarios are possible depending on the histology (CRC vs. SCC) and staging of the cancer, the IBD type, and the extension and severity of the inflammatory lesions. In case of CRC in patients with UC, combined multimodality neoadjuvant therapy seems to be contraindicated due to the high risk of severe bloody diarrhea, massive luminal bleeding, and even toxic megacolon (a condition with a mortality rate as high as 40%). For these patients, regardless of the extension and severity of the colonic inflammation, the only treatment indicated is total proctocolectomy, with abdominoperineal excision and terminal ileostomy. However, when the entire colon (and thus the UC target) is excised, the patient should undergo standard postoperative adjuvant treatment and radiotherapy. In case of CRC in a patient with CD limited to the distal colon and with sufficient control of mucosal inflammation, a proximal diverting colonostomy on the descending colon should be performed, with multimodality radio- and chemotherapy treatment initiated preoperatively. Otherwise, in case of severe inflammation, surgical resection must be the first therapeutic step. The most challenging condition is when CRC is diagnosed in a CD patient who has multiple concomitant strictures and/or inflammation in jejunoileal and colonic segments. The surgical intervention must be planned by considering, besides excision of the cancer, treatment of all CD locations, in order to minimize the risk of complications or CD recurrence during postoperative adjuvant therapy. Conservative surgery, such as minimal bowel resections and strictureplasties, is not recommended in these situations. This is an important topic considering that endoscopic recurrence of CD is detected at the site of the anastomosis within one year after resection in 73% of the patients [19]. The same considerations made for CRC are equally valid when a diagnosis of SCC is confirmed. However, due to the optimal response to multimodality neoadjuvant therapy and good prognosis of this cancer, a reasonable risk should be taken with respect to IBD-related complications.

8.4 Outcome

The outcome of patients with a cancer arising from a perianal fistula in IBD is difficult to standardize, and each case has its own history. In fact, the challenging diagnosis and staging of these cancers, and the consequent heterogeneity in treatment, lead to different results. In general, patients with CRC have a poor prognosis, with a mortality rate of 80-90% in 5 years and half of the patients will die within one year after the diagnosis. Patients with SCC have a better prognosis and when a neoadjuvant multimodality approach is feasible the 5-year survival rate is 45–55%, or even better for very early lesions [17].

8.5 Conclusions

Although cancer arising in perianal disease associated with IBD is rare, malignancy should be suspected in patients with persistent or new symptoms despite adequate treatment. Since very few data are available regarding both the primary treatment of cancer and the management of the underlying IBD, a tailored multidisciplinary approach, involving surgeons, gastroenterologists, radiologists, oncologists, and radiotherapists, is mandatory for the treatment of these complex cases.

References

1. Penner A, Crohn BB (1938) Perianal fistulae as a complication of regional ileitis. Ann Surg 108(5):867-873
2. Tang LY, Rawsthorne P, Bernstein CN (2006) Are perineal and luminal fistulas associated in Crohn's disease? A population-based study. Clin Gastroenterol Hepatol 4(9):1130-1134
3. Hellers G, Bergstrand O, Ewerth S, Holmstrom B (1980) Occurrence and outcome after primary treatment of anal fistulae in Crohn's disease. Gut 21:525-527
4. Schwartz DA, Loftus EV, Tremaine WJ, et al (2002) The natural history of fistulizing Crohn's disease in Olmsted County, Minnesota. Gastroenterology 122:875-880
5. Hamzaoglu I, Hodin RA (2005) Perianal problems in patients with ulcerative colitis. Inflamm Bowel Dis 11:856-859
6. Eaden JA, Abrams KR, Mayberry JF (2001) The risk of colorectal cancer in ulcerative colitis: a meta-analysis. Gut 48:526-535
7. Gyde SN, Prior P, Macartney JC, Thompson H, Waterhouse JA, Allan RN (1980) Malignancy in Crohn's disease. Gut 21(12):1024-1029
8. Canavan C, Abrams KR, Mayberry J (2006) Meta-analysis: colorectal and small bowel cancer risk in patients with Crohn's disease. Aliment Pharmacol Ther 23:1097-1104
9. Slater G, Greenstein A, Aufses AH Jr (1984) Anal carcinoma in patients with Crohn's disease. Ann Surg 199(3):348-350
10. Ky A, Sohn N, Weinstein MA, Korelitz BI (1998) Carcinoma arising in anorectal fistulas of Crohn's disease. Dis Colon Rectum 41(8):992-996
11. Gilbert JM, Mann CV, Scholefield J, Domizio P (1991) The aetiology and surgery of carcinoma of the anus, rectum and sigmoid colon in Crohn's disease. Negative correlation with human papillomavirus type 16 (HPV 16). Eur J Surg Oncol 17(5):507-513
12. Ficari F, Fazi M, Garcea A, Nesi G, Tonelli F (2005) Anal carcinoma occurring in Crohn's disease patients with chronic anal fistula. Suppl Tumori 4(3):S31
13. Van Assche G, Dignass A, Reinisch W, et al (2010) The second European evidence-based Consensus on the diagnosis and management of Crohn's disease: Special situations. J Crohn Colitis 4:63-101
14. Haggett PJ, Moore NR, Shearman JD, Travis SPL, Jewell DP, Mortensen NJ (1995) Pelvic and perineal complications of Crohn's disease: assessment using magnetic resonance imaging. Gut 36:407-410
15. Sloots CE, Felt-Bersma RJ, Poen AC, Cuesta MA, Meuwissen SGM (2001) Assessment and classification of fistula-in-ano in patients with Crohn's disease by hydrogen peroxide enhanced transanal ultrasound. Int J Colorectal Dis 16:292-297
16. Orsoni P, Barthet M, Portie F, et al (1999) Prospective comparison of endosonography, magnetic resonance imaging and surgical findings in anorectal fistula and abscess complicating Crohn's disease. Br J Surg 86:360-4
17. Thomas M, Bienkowski R, Vandermeer TJ, Trostle D, Cagir B (2010) Malignant transformation in perianal fistulas of Crohn's disease: a systematic review of the literature. J Gastrointest Surg 14:66-73
18. Goessling W, Mayer RJ (2006) Systemic treatment of patients who have colorectal cancer and inflammatory bowel disease. Gastroenterol Clin North Am 35:714-727
19. Rutgeerts P, Geboes K, Vantrappen G, Beyls J, Kerremans R, Hiele M (1990) Predictability of the postoperative course of Crohn's disease. Gastroenterology 99: 956-963

Section III

Clinical Examination and Medical Needs

Clinical Examination 9

Andrea Bondurri, Piergiorgio Danelli and Matteo Marone

9.1 Introduction

Anamnesis and clinical examination are the basis of a thorough and effective approach to a patient with coloproctological disease and must be performed in an environment that is comfortable for him or her. In this type of examination, embarrassment concerning the nature of the problem is added to the usual "white-coat-induced stress." Embarrassment may be directly related to symptoms or to the strict association of the symptoms with genital or urinary function. Therefore, the physician must be sensitive when asking the patient about symptoms, following a pattern that allows evacuation habits, problem in urinary and fecal continence, and sexual problems to be sequentially addressed. Adequate patient preparation will allow a satisfactory endoscopic evaluation.

The physician's office should be divided into two different rooms, a comfortable room for anamnesis and another room for the physical examination (Figs. 9.1, 9.2). The patient's history has to be fully noted, including past medical history and pharmacological therapy as well as current problems. Since the clinical examination is unpleasant for the patient, we recommend that the entire procedure be explained to the patient in advance in order to improve collaboration.

A complete physical examination must always be performed. Abdominal tenderness, hepatomegaly, splenomegaly, groin adenopathy, should be identified and described. In a patient with Crohn's disease, abdominal masses can be a sign of ileal dilatation, intra-abdominal abscess, or mesenteric adenopathy. In such patients, enterocutaneous fistula or multiple abdominal scars can be

A. Bondurri (✉)
General Surgery 1, Luigi Sacco University Hospital
Milan, Italy
e-mail: bondurri.andrea@hsacco.it

M.Tonolini and G. Maconi (eds.), *Imaging of Perianal Inflammatory Diseases*,
DOI: 10.1007/978-88-470-2847-0_9, © Springer-Verlag Italia 2013

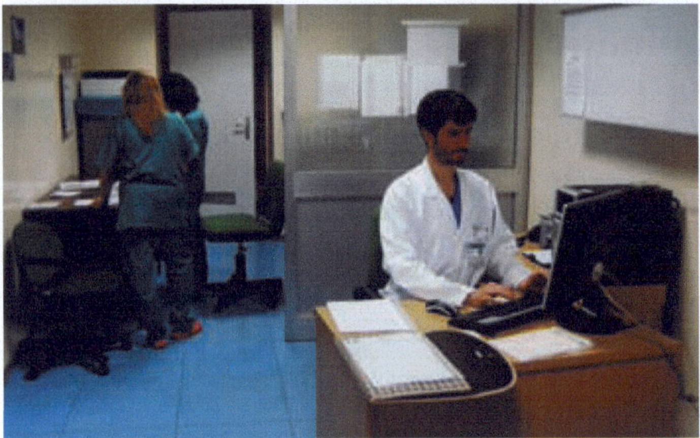

Fig. 9.1 Anamnesis room

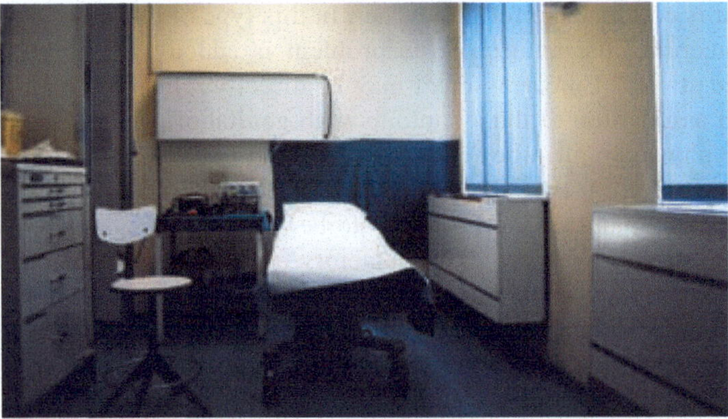

Fig. 9.2 Physical examination room

observed. Any doubt during the clinical exam should be pursued with the proper imaging test.

The perineal exam is based on three steps:

- Inspection and palpation of the perianal skin
- Digital exploration
- Examination of muscular function

The patient can be placed in different positions so as to facilitate the examination:

- Sim's position: The patient lies on his or her left side with the buttocks near the edge of the examination table and knees in flexion (Fig. 9.3).

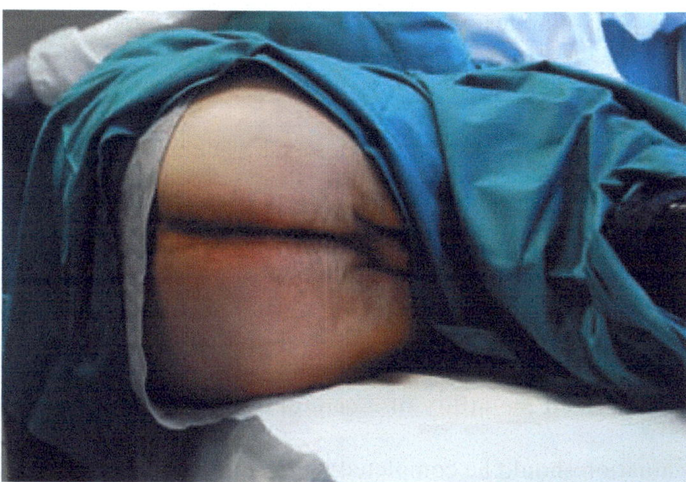

Fig 9.3 Sim's position

- Lithotomy position: The patient lies supine, with the perineum positioned at the edge of the examination table and the feet above or at the same level as the hips.
- Prone knee-chest position: This allows a better visualization of the rectum, although it is very uncomfortable for the patient.
- Prone jack-knife position: This requires a special table and allows an optimal view of the anterior rectal wall [2].

The inspection begins with an examination of the perianal skin, looking for a fistula orifice, excoriation, hemorrhoids, swelling, scars, vegetations, prolapses, and skin disease. The examiner should ask the patient to bear down, which allows the presence of rectal prolapse and the proper descent of the perineum, usually to a level about 10 mm above the ischial tuberosity, to be determined.

Palpation consists of applying firm pressure on both the ischial tuberosity and the skin around the anal orifice, in order to detect fistula or abscess. During this part of the examination, the anal reflex (L1–L2) can be evoked with a rounded pin.

During digital exploration, the examiner's well lubricated, gloved index finger is inserted in the patient's rectum and the rectal circumference is checked, searching for the presence of masses, tenderness, hemorrhoids, ulcers, fistula tracts, secretions, and pain triggers. The examiner first softly presses the perianal skin and then introduces his or her index finger into the rectum, in the direction of the navel. This part of the examination has two important considerations: (1) the exploration must be performed 1–2 cm after the anal orifice and (2) the whole index finger must be inserted.

The presence of a particular lesion has to be described, referring to its dimension, consistency, shape, fixity, tenderness, ulceration. Clearly, it is also very important to describe where the lesion is located, using the clock face system of description.

In a patient with inflammatory bowel disease, rectal examination may not be possible due to anal canal stenosis. In such cases, evaluation under anesthesia should be performed.

Muscular function can be evaluated during the rectal exploration as well, by again asking the patient to bear down, during which the normal contraction of the anal sphincter is determined. Correct abdominal wall muscle recruitment, which usually allows defecation through the Valsalva maneuver, is confirmed. While anorectal tests are necessary to diagnose defecatory disorders, recent studies have highlighted the utility of a careful digital rectal examination [1, 3].

Every clinical evaluation should be completed with anoscopy or rigid proctosigmoidoscopy.

References

1. Pescatori M (2011) Ascessi, fistole anali e retto vaginali. Springer, Milan
2. Corman M (2005) Colon & rectal surgery 5th edn. Lippincot Williams & Wilkins, Philadelphia, pp. 7-27, 279-332
3. Bharucha AE (2011) Recent advances in functional anorectal disorders. Curr Gastroenterol Rep 13(4):316-322

Surgical Examination Under Anesthesia 10

Michele Crespi, Francesco Colombo and Diego Foschi

10.1 Introduction

In patients with Crohn's disease, the risk of developing a perineal complication (abscess and/or fistula) is very high (20–40 %) [1]. The presence of a fistula and/or abscess is associated with significant morbidity, which may include frequent hospitalization, surgical treatments, and a risk of incontinence. It is therefore mandatory to perform a complete clinical and instrumental evaluation of these patients, to identify all perianal abscesses and/or fistulas.

10.2 Initial Diagnostic Approach

After an accurate perianal examination, several second-line diagnostic tools [2] are available:

1. Magnetic resonance imaging (MRI) should be the initial procedure, as it is precise and non-invasive. It is not routinely necessary for patients with simple fistulas (European Crohn's and Colitis Organisation (ECCO) statement 9 A, 2010).
2. Examination under anesthesia (EUA) is the gold standard. It is most sensitive only when carried out by an experienced surgeon (ECCO statement 9 B, 2010) [3, 4].
3. Endoscopic ultrasound (EUS) is equivalent to pelvic MRI if rectal stenosis has been excluded (ECCO statement 9 C, 2010).

M. Crespi (✉)
Department of Surgery, Gastroenterology and Oncology, Luigi Sacco University Hospital
Milan, Italy
e-mail: crespi.michele@hsacco.it

M.Tonolini and G. Maconi (eds.), *Imaging of Perianal Inflammatory Diseases*,
DOI: 10.1007/978-88-470-2847-0_10, © Springer-Verlag Italia 2013

4. Proctosigmoidoscopy should be used routinely in the initial evaluation (ECCO statement 9 D, 2010).

With the combination of two of these diagnostic modalities (MRI + EUA or EUA +EUS), an accuracy of 100% can be reached [5] (evidence-based medicine level IIb).

The gold standard in the evaluation of perianal disease is EUA, which is a very sensitive procedure (accuracy of 90% in the hands of an expert surgeon) [6]. Furthermore EUA is fundamental for the diagnosis and classification of abscesses and fistulas.

In the operating room, EUA allows abscess drainage (to prevent local injury due to undrained sepsis) and fistula treatment via fistulectomy/fistulotomy or with seton placement. Another important aspect of EUA is that in a large number of patients with perianal Crohn's disease a complete clinical evaluation in the ambulatory setting is simply not possible.

10.3 Classification of Anal Fistulas

Anal fistulas are classified according to the system described by Parks et al. [12] (Fig. 10.1):

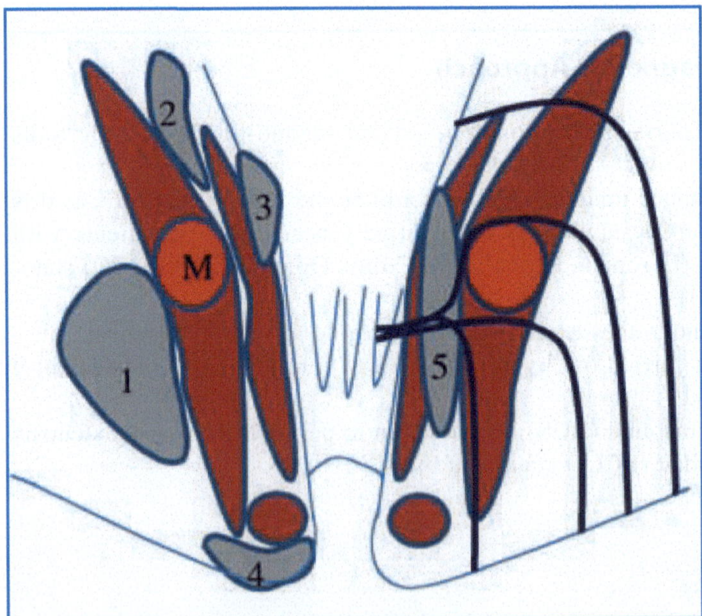

Fig. 10.1 Parks classification of anal fistulas and abscesses *1* Ischiorectal abscess, *2* supralevator abscess, *3* submucosal abscess, *4* perianal abscess, *5* intersphincteric abscess, *M* puborectalis muscle

- Type I: Intersphincteric fistula
- Type II: Transsphincteric fistula
- Type III: Suprasphincteric fistula
- Type IV: Extrasphincteric fistula.

The American Gastroenterological Association (AGA) proposed a simpler classification system for fistulas, comprising two groups, simple and complex [7]:

1. Simple fistulas (low fistulas)
   a. Superficial, low intersphincteric, low intrasphincteric
   b. Single external opening
   c. No perianal abscess
   d. No connection with the vagina or bladder
   e. No rectal stenosis or macroscopic proctitis.

2. Complex fistulas (high fistulas)
   a. High intersphincteric, high intrasphincteric, suprasphincteric, extrasphincteric
   b. Several external openings
   c. Perianal abscess
   d. Connection with the bladder or vagina
   e. Rectal stenosis or macroscopic proctitis.

10.4 Surgical Principles of EUA

In carrying out EUA, the following surgical instruments are needed (Fig. 10.2):
- Anal retractor
- Vaginal speculum
- Probe and setons
- Syringe
- Methylene blue or H_2O_2
- Anoscope

Note that it is very important to obtain an extensive informed consent from the patient, because EUA potentially comprises several different surgical procedures.

10.4.1 Physical Examination

The main aim of a correct perianal examination is to achieve a proper diagnosis and to classify all the abscesses and fistulas, to avoid missing hidden conditions. The surgeon should thoroughly evaluate the perineum, looking for an external opening of the fistula and spontaneous discharges from its orifices. A digital rectal exploration may lead to the detection of fibrotic tissue under the skin, representing the fistula tract, which may also be noted

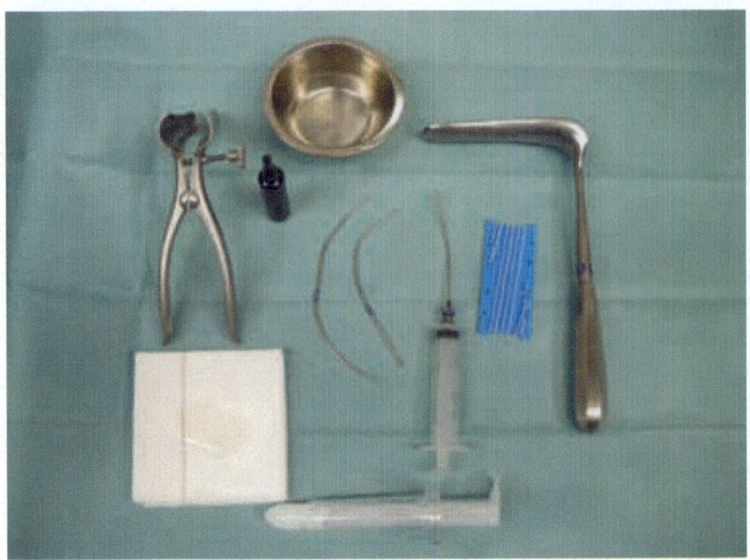

Fig. 10.2 Surgical instruments of EUA

as an induration of the perianal tissue. As discussed above, physical examination allows definition of the type of fistula, according to either the Parks or the AGA classification, and the detection of any connections with the vagina.

Both the anal retractor and the vaginal speculum can be very useful to identify the fistula's internal orifice (Figs. 10.3, 10.4).

A standard probing exploration (Fig. 10.5) is mandatory to confirm the type of fistula, to identify internal orifices, and to assess the involvement of the anal sphincters. The syringe-injection of methylene blue or H_2O_2 (Fig. 10.6) through the orifices of the fistula will in most cases highlight the different tracts in complex fistulas.

Abscess drainage is essential to prevent diffuse sepsis, to avoid sphincter injuries, and to treat local symptoms. In patients with Crohn's disease and those with inflammatory bowel diseases in general, an EUA is very important in efforts to resolve local inflammation/infection in patients who are candidates for medical treatment.

10.4.2 Fistula Treatment

Treatment options during EUA include the following:

- Fistulotomy of simple fistulas (AGA classification): healing rate of 75–85% [8]

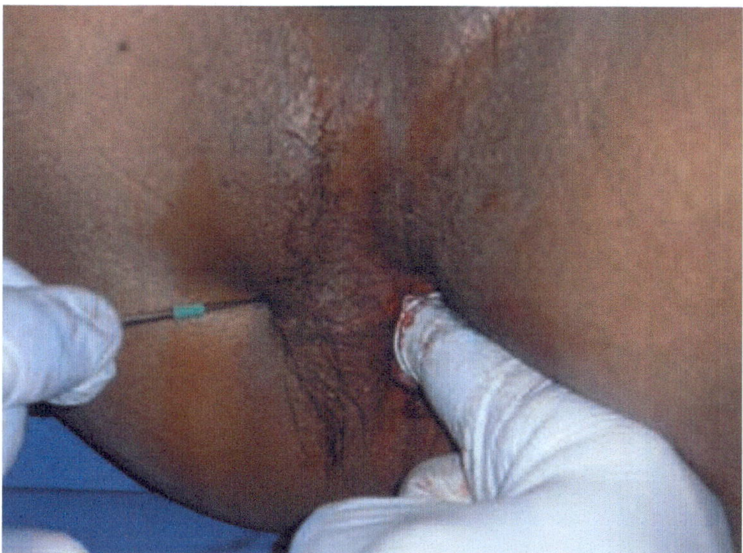

Fig. 10.3 Perianal examination, including the external orifice of a fistula

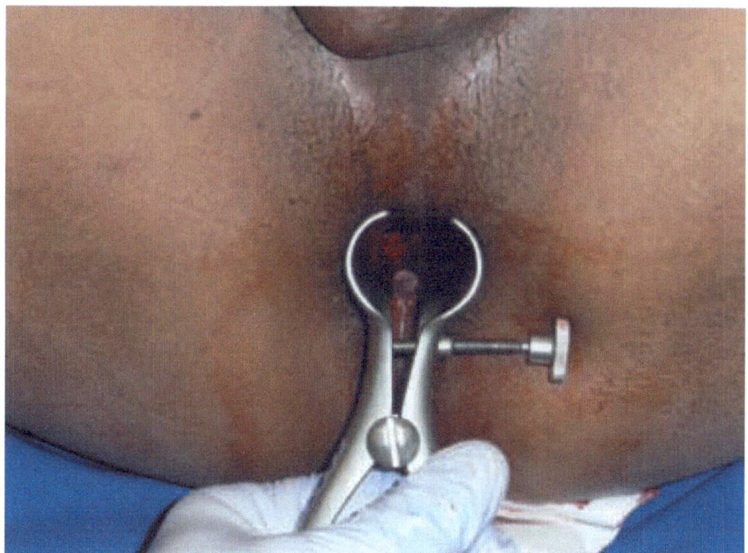

Fig. 10.4 Exploration of the anal canal with the anoscope

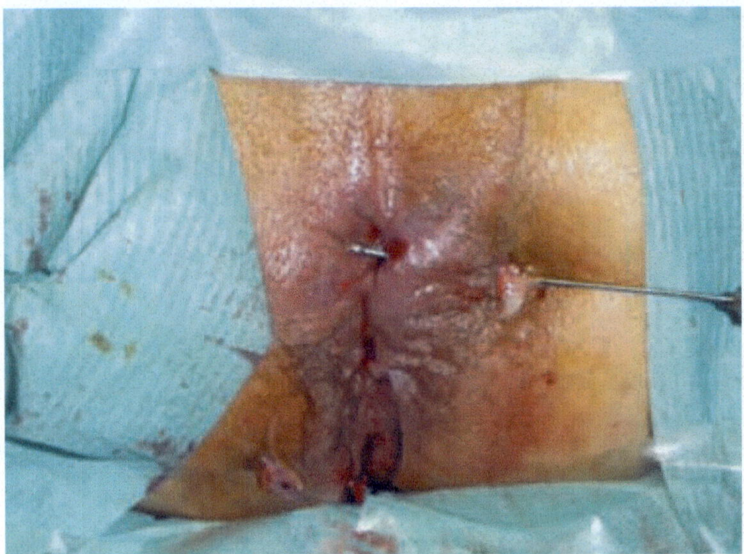

Fig. 10.5 Probing exploration in a complex fistula

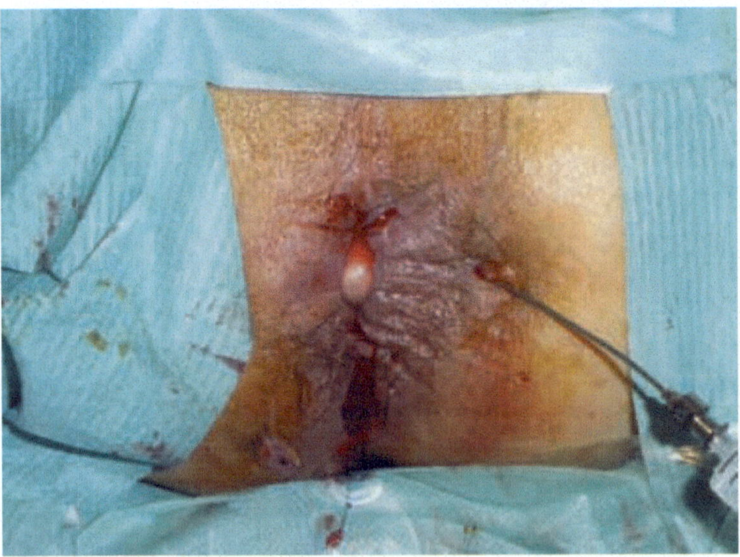

Fig. 10.6 Probing exploration with H_2O_2

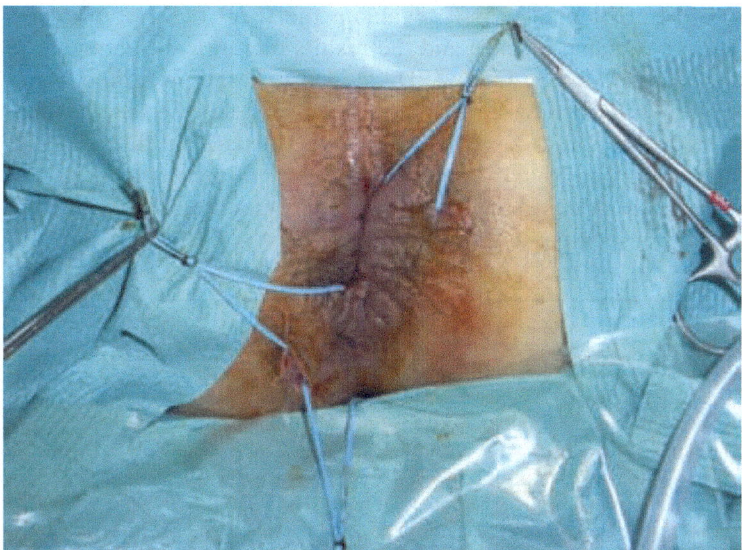

Fig. 10.7 Placement of a non-cutting setons in a complex fistula

- Fistulectomy of an extrasphincteric fistula tract
- Placement of non-cutting setons in complex fistulas or to treat active rectal disease (AGA classification) (Fig. 10.7). A loose seton prevents abscess formation and facilitates drainage of the fistula [9, 10].

10.4.3 Follow-Up

In patients with complex perianal Crohn's disease, follow-up with EUA [8] is essential, mostly to reassess the local situation and to evaluate the correct timing of seton removal (a seton is rarely curative!).

Reports in the most recent literature recommend endoanal ultrasound prior to and after EUA to accurately identify perianal disease and in follow-up of the surgical procedure [11].

10.5 Reassessment After Surgery

According to the guidelines of the European Medicines Agency, in the management of fistulizing Crohn's disease the goals of therapy are to close the fistula and maintain its closure, to reduce the need for surgical interventions, and to maintain the fistula in a closed state while avoiding the development of new fistulas.

There are two different measures to evaluate the level of discomfort of patients with Crohn's perianal disease and the results of surgical treatments:

- The Perineal Disease Activity Index (PDAI) measures the morbidity associated with perianal disease based on five categories related to the fistula: discharge, pain, restriction of sexual activity, type of perianal disease, and degree of induration. The PDAI is very useful in the clinical setting.
- The Fistula Drainage Assessment assesses fistula closure, defined as no drainage for two consecutive assessments for at least 4 weeks.

References

1. Schwartz D, Loftus E, Tremaine W, Panaccione R, Sandborrn W (2000) The natural history of fistulizing Crohn's disease: a population based study. Gastroenterology 118;A337
2. Van Assche G, Dignass A, Reinsch w, et al for the European Crohn's and Colitis Organisation (ECCO) (2010) The secod European evidence-based Consensus on the diagnosis and management of Crohn's disease: special situations. J Crohn's Colitis 4, 63–101
3. Schwartz DA, Loftus EV, Tremaine WJ, et al (2002) The natural history of fistulizing Crohn's disease in Olmsted County, Minnesota. Gastroenterology 122:875–80
4. Tang LY, Rawsthorne P, Bernstein CN (2006) Are perineal and luminal fistulas associated in Crohn's disease? A population-based study. Clin Gastroenterol Hepatol 4:1130–4
5. Schwartz DA, Wiersema MJ, Dudiak KM et al (2001) A comparison of endoscopic ultrasound, magnetic resonance imaging, and examination under anaesthesia for evaluation of Crohn's perianal fistulas. Gastroenterology 121:1064-1072
6. Taxonera C, Schwartz DA, García-Olmo D (2009) Emerging treatments for complex perianal fistula in Crohn's disease. World J Gastroenterol 15(34): 4263-4272
7. American Gastroenterological Association (2003) Medical position statement: perianal Crohn's disease. Gastroenterology 125: 1503-1507
8. Lodberg Hvas C, Dhlerup JF el al (2010) Diagnosis and treatment of fistulising Crohn's disease. Clinical guidelines. Danish Medical Bulletin Dec 58(10): C4338
9. Faucheron JL, Saint-Marc O, Guibert L et al (1996) Long term seton drainage for high anal fistula in Crohn's disease. A sphincter saving operation ?. Dis Colon Rectum 39: 208-211
10. Duff S, Sagar P, Rao M, et al (2012) Infliximab and surgical treatment of complex anal Crohn's disease. Colorectal Disease 14:972-976
11. Tilney HS, Heriot AG, Trickett JP el al (2006) The use of intra-operative endo-anal ultrasound in perianal disease. Colorectal Dis 8(4): 338-41
12. Parks AG, Gordon PH, Hardcastle JD (1976) A classification of fistula-in-ano. Br J Surg; 63(1):1-12

Section IV

Ultrasound

Techniques 11

Elisa Radice, Giovanni Maconi and Giulio A. Santoro

11.1 Transanal Ultrasound

Transanal ultrasound was the first technique used to directly depict the anal sphincter complex in detail. It requires a high-frequency transducer for detailed resolution, near-field focusing, and an axial 360° image to view circular sphincteric structures [1]. This is possible with a mechanically rotated single crystal, although it is a technology now considered obsolete by the majority of ultrasound manufacturers. The system uses a hard plastic cone to protect the rotating endoprobe. The outer walls of this cone are parallel, so that the probe may be moved within the anal canal without causing any anatomical distortion.

The transanal ultrasound examination is easy to perform, minimally invasive, and well tolerated by the patient as it requires no bowel preparation. The patients are usually examined in the left lateral or prone position, since either one yields a highly accurate view of the anterior aspect of the external sphincter and perineum. The dynamic nature of the investigation allows the patient's position to be changed in order to optimize the visualization of anorectal structures. In two-dimensional (2D) ultrasound, the probe is gently inserted into the distal rectum and then withdrawn through the anal canal. After it reaches the ampulla, the operator must look for the rectovaginal septum in females and the prostate in males. As the probe is withdrawn, the urethra may be seen anteriorly (Fig. 11.1). At the origin of the anal canal, the U-shaped sling of the puborectalis muscle is the main landmark and should be used for anal adjustment of the probe. The internal sphincter is visualized as a hypoechoic ring encir-

G. Maconi (✉)
Gastroenterology Unit, Department of Biomedical and Clinical Sciences
Luigi Sacco University Hospital
Milan, Italy
e-mail: giovanni.maconi@unimi.it

M.Tonolini and G. Maconi (eds.), *Imaging of Perianal Inflammatory Diseases*,
DOI: 10.1007/978-88-470-2847-0_11,

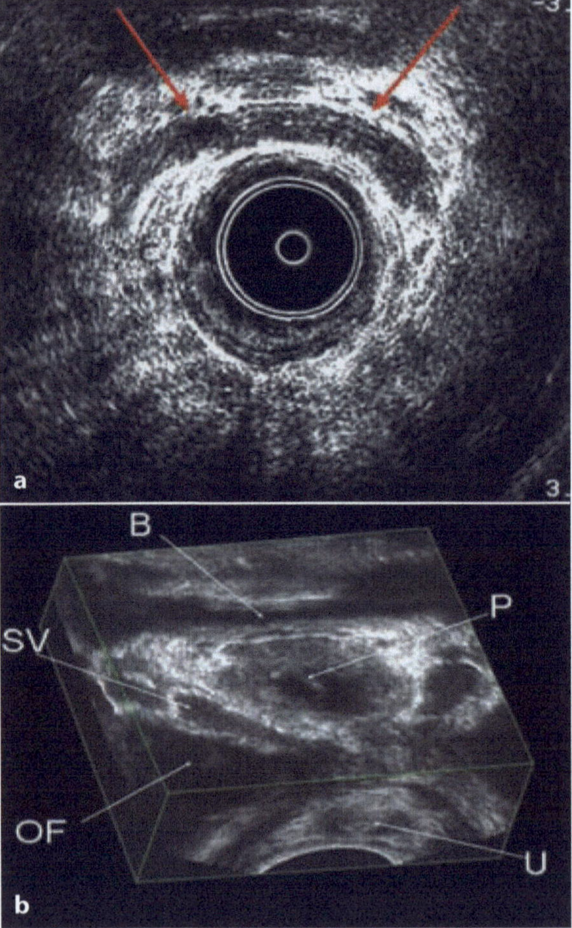

Fig. 11.1 Orientation of the rectal probe. The probe is placed in the distal part of the ampulla; the anterior side is indicated by the vagina (*arrows*) and rectovaginal septum in women (**a**) and by the prostate (*P*) in men (**b**). In this 3D scan, the seminal vesicle (*SV*), urethra (*U*), and bladder (*B*) are seen anteriorly

cling the anal canal, whereas the external sphincter is of mixed echogenicity. The intersphincteric space and longitudinal muscle lie between these structures and are of mixed echogenicity (Fig. 11.2).

The investigation takes only a few minutes. Probes of several frequencies are available, from 2.5 to 16 MHz. The latter is preferably used to image the anal and rectal walls and the internal sphincter in particular, while the former allows the investigation of deeper lesions such as in the perirectal and perianal spaces. However, despite the value of 2D transanal ultrasound, it has several shortcomings. Images are normally produced only in the transaxial scanning plane. Scanning in the proximal-distal direction can be extended only by moving the probe further in or out of the anal canal or rectum.

Nowadays, it has become possible to obtain three-dimensional (3D) reconstructions of 2D images, which has vastly improved the usefulness and accu-

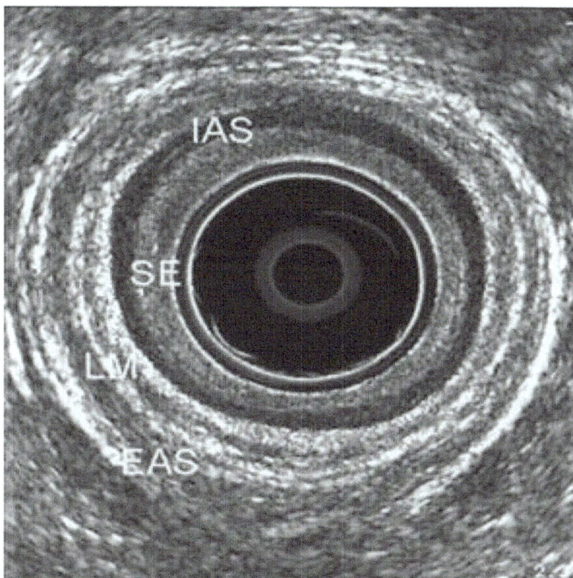

Fig. 11.2 The anal sphincter complex at transanal ultrasound. The internal anal sphincter (*IAS*) appears as a hypoechoic ring and the external anal sphincter (*EAS*) as a tissue of mixed echogenicity, with longitudinal muscle (*LM*) between them. *SE* subepithelial tissue

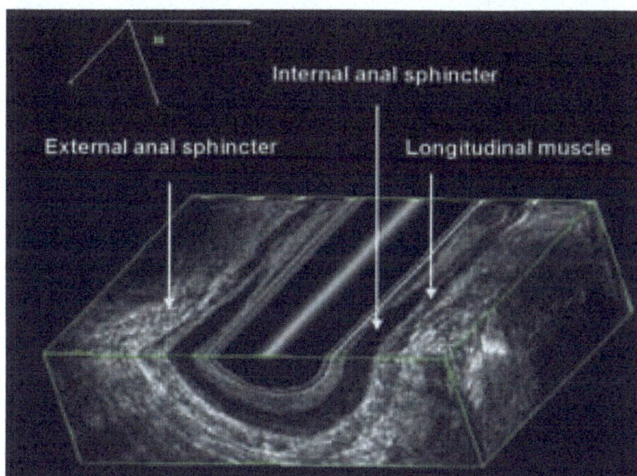

Fig. 11.3 A 3D transanal ultrasound reconstruction of the normal anorectal junction. Courtesy of Prof. Giulio A. Santoro, from [11]

racy of anal endosonography [2]. With this technique, data from a series of closely spaced 2D images are combined to create a 3D image that can be freely rotated and sliced to allow the operator to extract the most information out of the data—freed from the time pressure of the examination itself. After a data set is acquired, coronal anterior–posterior (A–P) or posterior–anterior (P–A) as well as sagittal right–left (R–L) views can be selected (Fig. 11.3). The same endoprobe and multifrequency transducers used in 2D transanal ultrasound are also used in the 3D method. A 3D reconstruction is based on a large number of parallel transaxial images acquired using a special colorectal pullback mover (B&K Medical ultrasound probe type 1850). The B&K Medical pullback mover can be operated at different levels of resolution. For endoanal applications, the usual setting is 0.2–0.3 mm between adjacent transaxial images. Scanning the anal canal with these settings over a pullback distance of 35 mm typically yields 175 parallel images. These views constitute a source of information with which to further evaluate the patient. In patients with perianal fistula, both the fistula type and the extent of anal sphincter damage can be seen. The diagnosis is less dependent on one examiner, because the data can be reviewed by several specialists.

Finally, the latest development is the combined use of 3D transanal ultrasound and hydrogen peroxide. If an external opening of the fistula can be identified, a flexible intravenous cannula (e.g., Venflon) can be used to introduce hydrogen peroxide into the opening immediately before a 3D data set is acquired [3], which allows better visualization of the fistulous tract. Data acquisition takes approximately 40 s for a high-resolution scan. During this

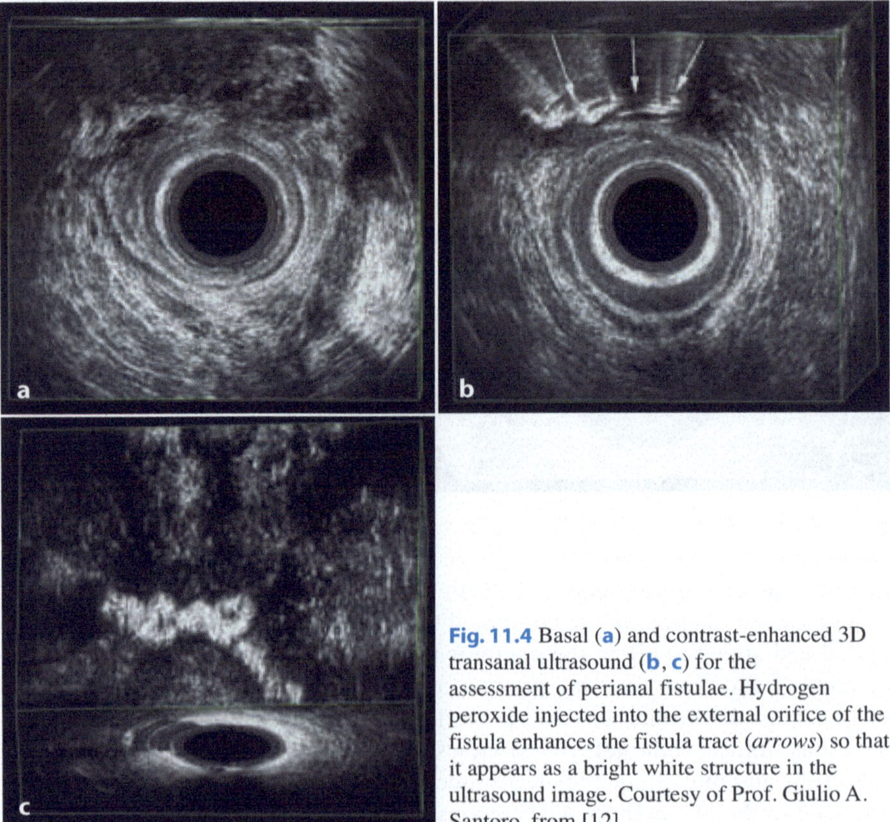

Fig. 11.4 Basal (**a**) and contrast-enhanced 3D transanal ultrasound (**b**, **c**) for the assessment of perianal fistulae. Hydrogen peroxide injected into the external orifice of the fistula enhances the fistula tract (*arrows*) so that it appears as a bright white structure in the ultrasound image. Courtesy of Prof. Giulio A. Santoro, from [12]

short period, the hydrogen peroxide enhances the fistula tract so that it appears as a bright white structure in the ultrasound image (Fig. 11.4). Aerated and diluted lidocaine gel may also be introduced into an external opening as an ultrasound-enhancing medium. This technique is a safe, economic, and reliable procedure for the assessment of perianal fistulae [3-6]. It assists in delineating their anatomic course and is therefore of value in the planning of surgical strategies.

11.2 Transperineal Ultrasound

Despite the advantages of its high-resolution and versatility in the study of the anal canal, transanal ultrasound has several limitations in the assessment of perianal inflammatory disease since pain experienced by the patient may restrict transducer placement. Moreover, the rigid probe, positioned within the anal canal or rectum, may be inappropriately located for the assessment of the perianal soft tissues because the pathologic process, frequently involving the perineum and the buttocks, is either on a more caudal plane than or too far from the ultrasound beam.

Transperineal ultrasound has been proposed to overcome these limitations. In pregnant women [4] and in young children [5] it has been used to evaluate distal anorectal and perirectal abnormalities. It is generally well-tolerated and thus preferred by patients; in those cases in which it can provide equivalent information, it has the potential to replace transanal ultrasound.

Transperineal sonography is performed using the same transducers already found in most sonography practices. It shares several advantages with transanal ultrasound, such as its low-cost, high-resolution, multiplanarity, and real-time performance, but it has also two important limitations: (1) poor penetration below 5–6 cm and consequent inadequate visualization of tissues far from the probe, and (2) potential interference from air entrapped in cutaneous folds and protruding anal tumors. However, compared with transanal ultrasound, transperineal sonography has the advantage that it allows the visualization of perirectal and perineal processes several centimeters from the rectal lumen (enabled by multiple windows). Although the duration of the learning curve for this examination has not been determined, the required proficiency in evaluating the anal canal in male patients is substantial, while most experienced abdominal sonographers achieve competency after approximately 12 patients [7].

Transperineal sonography does not require specific preparation of the patient (i.e., enema or evacuation suppositories). In addition to 3.5- to 10-MHz microconvex or transvaginal arrays, linear, curved, or sectorial transducers operating at the highest frequency can be used. The probes are covered with gel and introduced into a latex examination glove or a condom, for hygienic reasons, that is covered with contact gel before the examination is performed. For the examination, the patient is placed in the dorsal lithotomy or left lateral position, after which the probe is positioned directly above the anus.

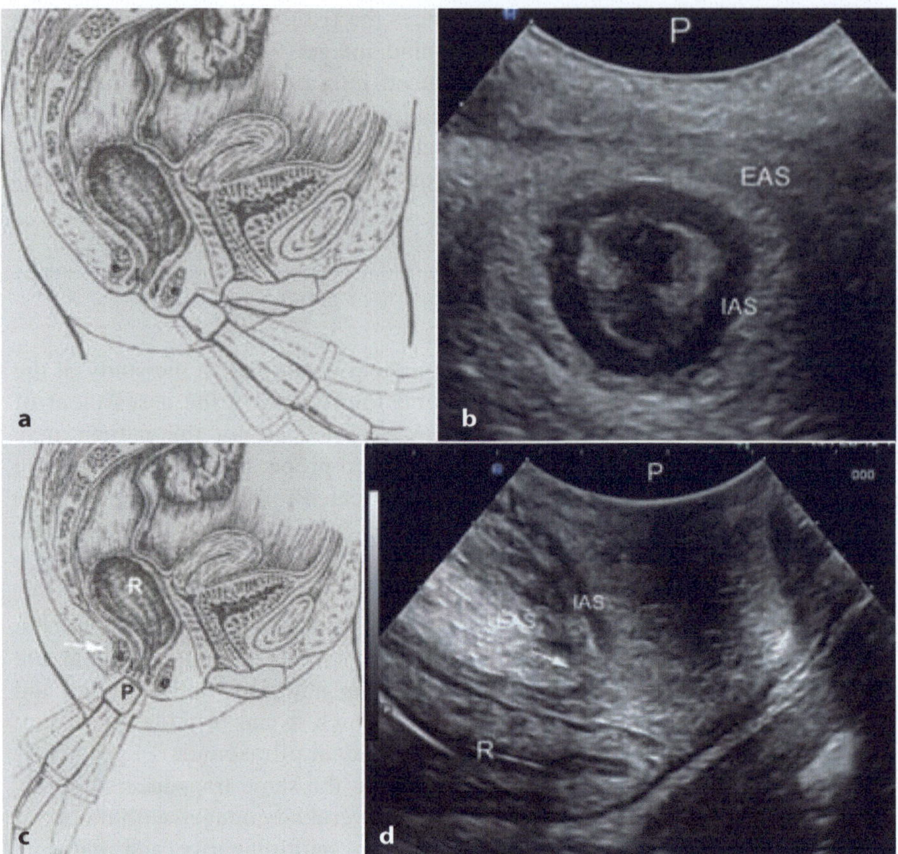

Fig. 11.5 Transperineal ultrasound. Technical approach (**a**, **c**) and correspondent findings (**b**, **d**). With the patient in the dorsal or left lateral position, the transducer is placed directly on the perineal body and then pressed posteriorly and angled craniocaudally to obtain a cross-sectional view, mainly in women (**a**, **b**); it can also be placed on the perineum to obtain a long axis view (**c**, **d**). In both sections, the internal anal sphincter (*IAS*) appears as a hypoechoic ring and the external anal sphincter (*EAS*) as a tissue of mixed echogenicity, as in anorectal ultrasound. *P* Probe, *R* rectum, *arrow* anorectal angle

Standard images are obtained from axial and longitudinal viewpoints on the perineal body, above the anus. Additional oblique images and angled images are obtained as needed to outline the anatomy and pathology of interest (Fig. 11.5). It is thereby possible to obtain high-resolution images of the anal canal, the anal sphincters, the puborectalis muscle, the rectovaginal and anovulvar septa, the urinary bladder, and the vagina. The internal anal sphincter is an approximately 3-mm-thick hypoechoic band completely surrounding the more echogenic rectal mucosa. The surrounding mixed-echogenicity striated external anal sphincter is slightly thicker, measuring approximately 5 mm [8-10].

References

1. Law PJ, Bartram CI (1989) Anal endosonography: technique and normal anatomy. Gastrointest Radiol 14:349–53
2. Santoro GA, Fortling B (2007) The advantages of volume rendering in three-dimensional endosonography of the anorectum. Dis Colon Rectum 50:359-68
3. West RL, Dwarkasing S, Schouten WR, et al (2004) Hydrogen peroxide-enhanced three-dimensional endoanal ultrasonography and endoanal magnetic resonance imaging in evaluating perianal fistulas: agreement and patient preference. Eur J Gastroenterol Hepatol 16:1319-24
4. Buchanan GN, Bartram CI, Williams AB, et al (2005) Value of hydrogen peroxide enhancement of three-dimensional endoanal ultrasound in fistula-in-ano. Dis Colon Rectum 48:141-7
5. Poen AC, Felt-Bersma RJ, Eijsbouts QA, et al (1998) Hydrogen peroxide-enhanced transanal ultrasound in the assessment of fistula-in-ano. Dis Colon Rectum 41:1147-52
6. Navarro-Luna A, Garcia-Domingo MI, Rius-Macias J, et al. (2004) Ultrasound study of anal fistulas with hydrogen peroxide enhancement. Dis Colon Rectum 47:108-14
7. Stewart LK, McGee J, Wilson SR (2001) Transperineal and transvaginal sonography of perianal inflammatory disease. AJR Am J Roentgenol 177:627-32
8. Hertzberg BS, Bowie ID, Weber TM, et al (1991) Sonography ofthe cervix during the third trimester of pregnancy: value of the transperineal approach. Am J Roentgenol 157:73-6
9. Teele RL, Share JC (1997) Transperineal sonography in children. Am J Roentgenol 168:1263-7
10. Campbell DM, Behan M, Donnelly VS, et al (1996) Endosonographic assessment of postpartum anal sphincter injury using a 120 degree sector scanner Clin Radiol 51:559-61
11. Santoro GA, Di Falco G (2004) Atlas of Endoanal and Endorectal Ultrasonography. Springer, Milan
12. Santoro GA, Wieczorek AP, Bartram CI (2010) Pelvic Floor Disorders. Springer, Milan

Crohn's Disease 12

Elisa Radice, Giovanni Maconi, Flavio Caprioli
and Guido Basilisco

12.1 Perianal Fistulas

Fistulization is one of the major troublesome issues of Crohn's disease (CD). Fistulas are abnormal tracts formed between the gut and the skin, between the gut and an abscess cavity, or between the gut and other hollow structures, including the vagina. Fistulas arises from ulcers that progress to deep transmural fissures which then eventually penetrate other structures or open into another organ. They are classified as internal or external depending on where they terminate. Internal fistulas are enteroenteric, gastrocolic, enterovaginal, and enterovescical; external fistulas are enterocutaneous, colocutaneous, or perianal.

The prevalence of fistulas in referral populations varies from 17 to 43%, and it has been estimated that 25–50% of patients with CD will develop a perianal fistula during the course of their disease. In a population-based study of the cumulative incidence of all types of CD fistulas, anovaginal or rectovaginal fistulas accounted for 9% [2–5]. The risk for developing a perianal fistula is higher in patients with CD involving the left colon and rectum.

Both perianal and rectovaginal fistulas can result in significant morbidity, related to acute abscesses, chronic discharge, low-grade sepsis, anal stenosis, or fecal incontinence. Accurate diagnosis is mandatory for the proper management of fistulas, since incorrect or inappropriate treatment may lead to irreversible functional consequences.

G. Maconi (✉)
Gastroenterology Unit, Department of Biomedical and Clinical Sciences
Luigi Sacco University Hospital
Milan, Italy
e-mail: giovanni.maconi@unimi.it

M.Tonolini and G. Maconi (eds.), *Imaging of Perianal Inflammatory Diseases*,
DOI: 10.1007/978-88-470-2847-0_12, © Springer-Verlag Italia 2013

12.2 Endoanal Sonography

12.2.1 Classification of Fistulas and Diagnostic Accuracy

The classification of perianal fistulas is mainly based upon their anatomical location. The simplest classification uses the dentate line as the reference point to classify fistulas as high (above the dentate line) or low (below the dentate line).

The most practical anatomical classification was proposed by Parks in 1976 [6], following an analysis of a surgical series of 400 patients and taking into account the relationship between the fistula and the anal sphincter complex. Four main types were identified: intersphincteric, transsphincteric, suprasphincteric, and extrasphincteric. Subsequently, a further superficial fistula, below the internal and external anal sphincters, was added.

The clinical classification proposed by the American Gastroenterological Association (AGA) distinguishes two main groups of fistulas: simple and complex [7, 11]. The simple fistula is low and therefore includes superficial, intersphincteric, and transsphincteric fistulas below the dentate line, fistulas with a single external orifice and lacking signs suggesting abscess, rectovaginal fistula, or rectal or anal stricture. A complex fistula is an intersphincteric, transsphincteric, suprasphincteric, or extrasphincteric fistula above the dentate line. It may have multiple external orifices or fluctuation suggesting an abscess. Complex fistulas include rectovaginal fistulas or an anal or rectal stricture (Fig. 12.1).

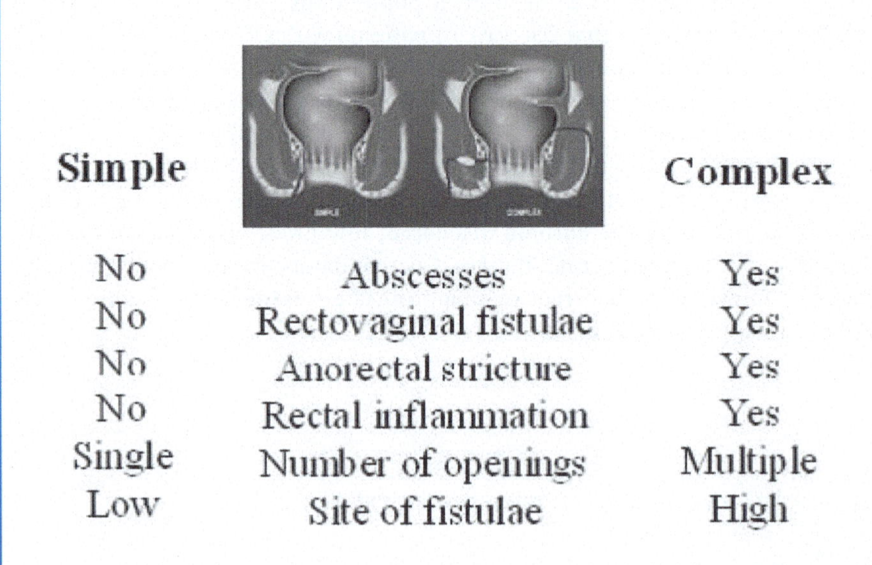

Fig. 12.1 American Gastroenterological Association classification of perianal disease

At transanal ultrasound, fistulous tracts may be identified as hypoechoic, round to oval structures that lie in any location within the anal wall. They can be internally hyperechoic (increased or bright echoes) if they contain gas. According to the Parks classification, intersphincteric fistulas are characterized by a primary tract that courses in the intersphincteric space without penetrating the external sphincter (Fig. 12.2). Transsphincteric fistulas traverse the external sphincter and pass into the ischianal fossa, below the level of the puborectalis muscle (Fig. 12.2). Suprasphincteric fistulas course within the intersphincteric plane superior to the puborectalis before penetrating the levator musculature to course within the ischiorectal and ischioanal fossae (Fig. 12.2). Extrasphincteric fistulas course within the ischioanal fossa and penetrate the levator musculature without traversing either the internal or the external sphincter, opening directly into the rectum (Fig. 12.2).

Besides the classification of fistulous tracts, it is important to report the site of the internal opening. This is very effectively identified by transanal ultrasound because the opening lies right at the probe surface. The opening may be detected as a gap or disruption of the mucosal integrity and is usually reported by describing the site (anterior, posterior, left, lateral), often using a clockface description (e.g., 12 o'clock anterior, 6 o'clock posterior, 3 o'clock left, 9 o'clock right lateral).

Along with the description of the primary fistula tract and the site of its internal opening, any branching, secondary tracts or areas of extension must be identified and reported. It is well known that missed extensions are the most

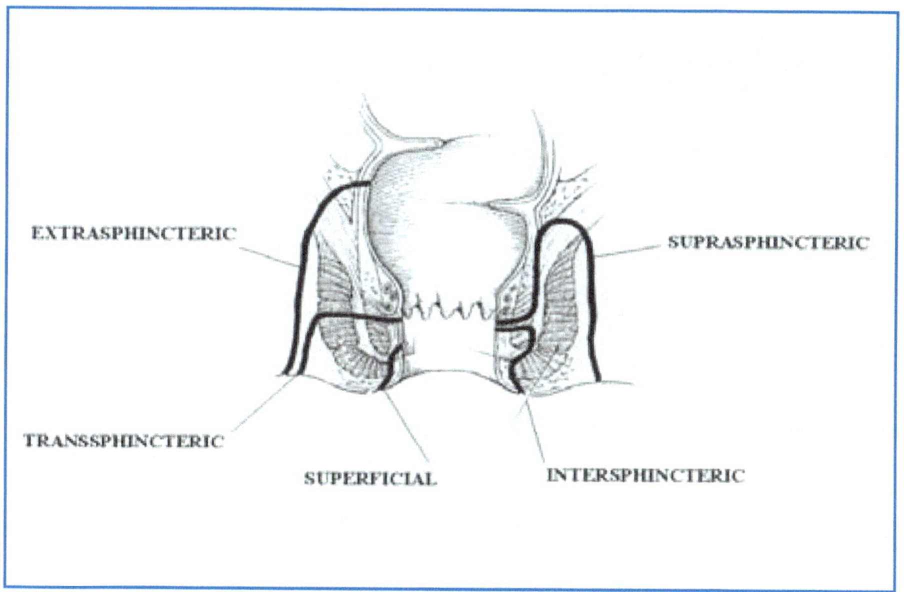

Fig. 12.2 The Parks classification of perianal fistulas

common cause of fistula recurrence after treatment [8]. Extensions may include blind-ending tracts and abscesses. These can be identified as an anechoic (without internal echoes) or hypoechoic mass (with internal echoes due to cellular debris or gas). When an abscess extends to either side of the internal opening it is described as a "horseshoe" abscess (Fig. 12.3). However, as transanal ultrasound is limited to the transversal plane, it is somewhat difficult to determine whether this extension is infralevator or supralevator. To overcome this difficulty and to improve the overall accuracy of transanal ultrasound, three-dimensional (3D) and contrast-enhanced ultrasound have been introduced. 3D transanal ultrasound is a volumetric acquisition of multiple parallel two-dimensional ultrasound images that are synthesized into a 3D data set, which may be manipulated digitally as an imaging volume. In contrast-enhanced transanal ultrasound a contrast agent, usually a 3% solution of hydrogen peroxide at a dose 2.5–5 ml, is injected before or during the examination into the external opening of a draining fistula, either directly using a syringe or by using a 16-G intravenous catheter connected by a short tube [9,10]. With this technique, perianal fistulas may be easily classified and the identification of extensions is both more accurate and simpler. However, it should be taken into account that this technique is feasible only in active draining fistulas. In patients with intermittent drainage, it may be difficult to introduce the catheter into the external orifice if it is temporarily closed. In this case, the patient should be examined without contrast agent and the contrast examination rescheduled. In addition, the passage of hydrogen peroxide into

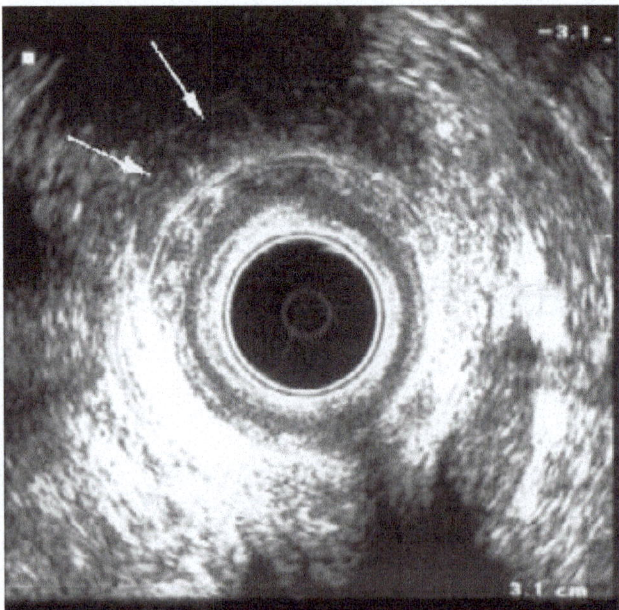

Fig. 12.3 Transanal ultrasound of the upper anal canal level in a male patient, showing a hypoechoic horseshoe extension well appreciable on the left side (*arrows*)

the lumen of the fistula may be slow or incomplete in fibrotic and inactive fistulas and may require an appropriate length of time to completely delineate the fistula and its extensions.

The accuracy of transanal ultrasound in evaluating CD perianal fistulas was assessed in several studies. A study from the Mayo Clinic [9] compared transanal ultrasound, magnetic resonance imaging (MRI), and surgical exploration under anesthesia (EUA), showing that more than one technique is required to fully describe and classify fistulas. In that study, 34 patients with suspected perianal fistulas were prospectively enrolled and their fistulas classified according to the Parks criteria. The accuracy of all three modalities was ≥85%: transanal ultrasound 91%, MRI 87%, and EUA 91%. However, accuracy was 100% when any two tests were combined.

The examination with contrast agent, especially when combined with 3D volumetric acquisition, has also proven to be superior to conventional ultrasound in demonstrating and delineating fistula tracts and in identifying internal fistula openings. A study investigating 41 patients with CD and perianal fistulas showed that a 3D contrast-enhanced examination can reveal a greater number of surgically difficult-to-treat fistulas (in up to 78% of patients, in the study) compared to conventional transanal ultrasound, suggesting that the technique is mandatory before surgery [10].

12.2.2 Assessment of Activity

Quantitative assessment of the activity of perianal fistulas in patients with CD may be of clinical relevance in disease management. Various clinical and instrumental methods are used for this purpose, such as fistula drainage assessment (FDA), the perianal disease activity index (PDAI), and MRI [12-16]. Transanal ultrasound also has been proposed for the assessment of perianal fistula activity. In general, active fistulas are visualized as intense hypoechoic tracts sometimes containing focal areas of hyperechogenicity consistent with gas bubbles, whereas inactive fistulas are visualized as less hypoechoic tracts lacking any hyperechoic foci [12, 14]. However, these ultrasonographic criteria in assessing fistula activity are limited by the visual ability to judge gray-scale echogenicity, which also may be influenced by the brightness and shadowing of surrounding structures. To overcome this limitation, Caprioli et al. suggested the quantitative computerized analysis of digitalized images of fistulas. The authors assessed fistula tract activity using both a subjective index and a computerized method. They found that active fistulas have a hypoechoic appearance that can be quantified by calculating the mean gray-scale tone [17]. According to the subjective index, the active fistula is described as a hypoechoic tract occasionally containing focal hyperechoic areas representing gas bubbles within, the inactive fistula is defined by the presence of less hypoechoic or isoechoic bands without any hyperechoic foci. The computerized method consists of the statistical image-analysis of gray-scale tones with-

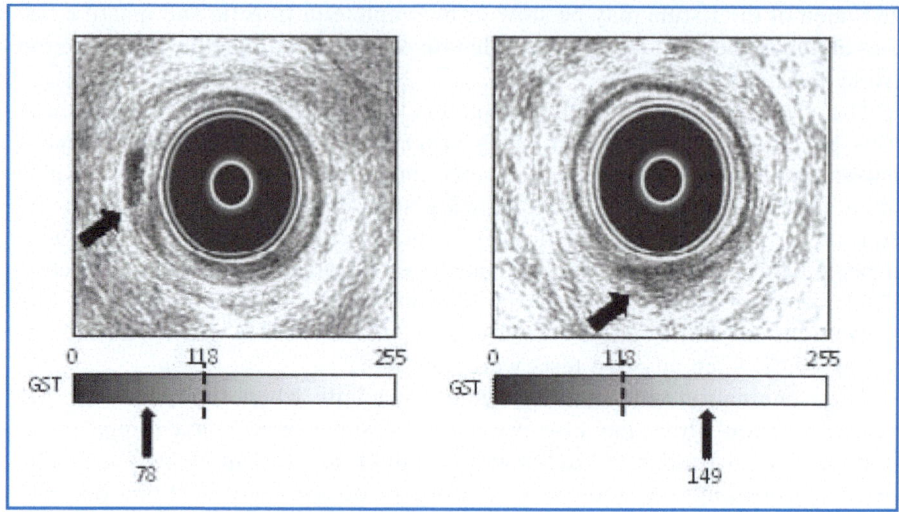

Fig. 12.4 Endosonogram of an active (*left*) and an inactive (*right*) perianal fistula, based on a gray-scale tone cut-off value discriminating active from inactive fistula. The overall gray-scale tone of the regions of interest taken at different levels of the fistula tract indicates the activity of the fistula

in a region of interest (ROI), as drawn using a computer mouse, on fistula tracts. This determination is assigned a number ranging from 0 (dark) to 255 (white) (Fig. 12.4). The authors showed that the agreement between clinical examination and transanal ultrasound was fair (k-value = 0.266-0.294), whereas that with computer-assisted analysis of anal ultrasound was good (k-value = 0.608-0.670) and quite similar to that between clinical examination and MRI (k-value = 0.739). These results were confirmed in another study by the same group, which showed that the gray-scale tone cut-off discriminating active from inactive fistula tracts is 117–118. It is worth noting that in the latter study transanal ultrasound was found to be complementary to other clinical scales and useful to assess perianal disease activity in CD [18]. Unfortunately, this method, although simple, is relatively time-consuming, unless specific software is integrated in the ultrasonographic device.

12.2.3 Follow-Up and Prognostic Findings

Over the last decade, anti-tumor necrosis factor-α (anti-TNF-α) antibodies (infliximab and adalimumab) have considerably improved the medical treatment of fistulizing CD. This class of drugs has proven to be an effective medical option for fistulizing CD, with a rate for the short-term cessation of fistula drainage > 65% [4]. However, both treatments also account for a high rate of abscess formation (up to 15%) due to premature closure of the cutaneous openings of the fistula tract [19]. Transanal ultrasound and MRI studies have demonstrated persistent fistula activity even after drainage of the fistula has stopped, resulting in a poor outcome. It is believed that the main reasons for fistula recurrence or abscess formation in perianal CD under treatment are fistula extensions or abscesses missed at the initial diagnostic work-up, premature cessation of therapy, or the premature removal of setons before the fistula has become inactive. Spradlin et al., in a prospective case-control study including five patients who received preoperative transanal ultrasound and five patients who did not, showed that transanal ultrasound at the initial preoperative diagnostic work-up demonstrates findings missed by initial EUA (in the control group), in their study specifically involving one patient with transsphincteric fistula and another with abscess. These occurrences resulted in further surgical interventions. The same study showed that seton removal while the fistula is still active can result in abscess or fistula formation due to premature closure of the cutaneous opening of the fistula [20].

These findings are in keeping with those of another study demonstrating the role of transanal ultrasound to monitor the effect of anti-TNF therapy in patients with perianal CD [21]. Infliximab is an effective treatment for fistulizing CD, yielding improvement or closure of the fistulous tracts. However, fistulas frequently re-open, suggesting the persistence of deep fistula tracts despite superficial healing. In this regard, we have shown that transanal ultrasound can detect the persistence of an internal active fistulous tract 10 weeks after anti-TNF treatment, despite closure of the fistula's external orifice, and that this condition poses a high risk of fistula relapse. By contrast, patients with closed perianal fistulas and disappearance of the fistula tract at transanal ultrasound have a significantly lower relapse rate [21].

These findings were confirmed by another study showing that regular transanal ultrasound may have an important role in defining patients with perianal fistulizing CD who could be treated (or re-treated) with infliximab and in identifying patients who can discontinue infliximab without recurrence of fistula drainage [22].

A further advantage of transanal ultrasound is its potential usefulness in guiding the puncture of an abscess [23]

12.3 Transperineal Ultrasound

Transperineal ultrasound is a simple, noninvasive and inexpensive technique to study the pelvis and perianal inflammatory diseases. It is an alternative to MRI or transanal ultrasound when, for various reasons, these procedures are contraindicated or not appropriate, in particular in children and in adults with anal strictures, painful perianal abscesses or lesions extending far from the anus and not accessible to transrectal ultrasound (e.g., gluteus or scrotum).

Several studies have shown that transperineal ultrasound can provide images of perianal fistulas comparable to those obtained with MRI (Fig. 12.5),

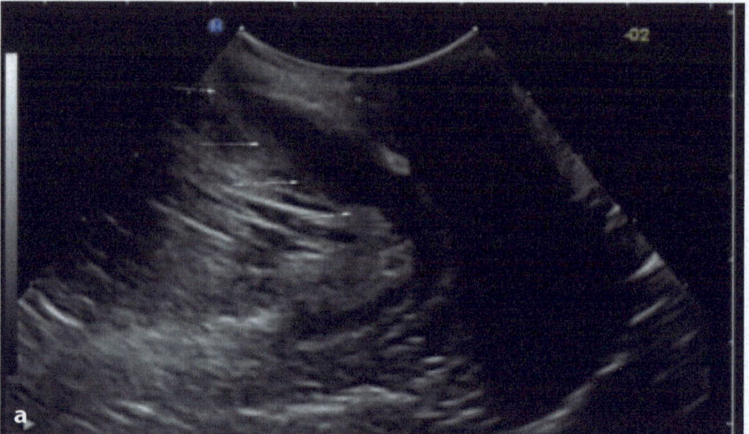

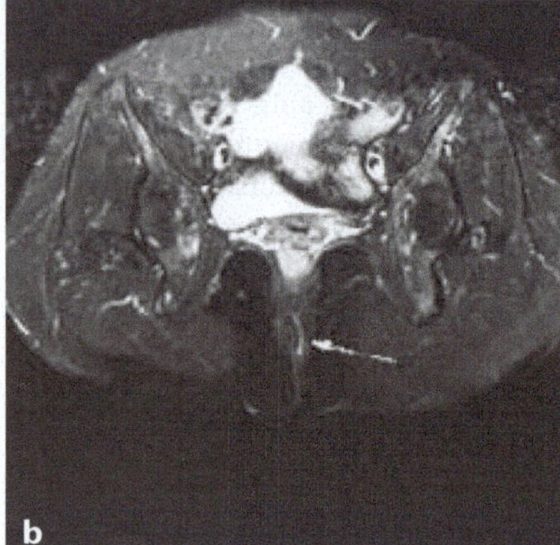

Fig. 12.5 Transsphincteric perianal fistula (*arrows*) assessed using transperineal ultrasound (**a**) and MRI in a T1 sequence with fat suppression (**b**)

and that its accuracy in detecting perianal fistulas and abscesses is comparable to that of MRI, transanal ultrasound, and surgical examination [24-27]. At ultrasound fistulas appear as hypoechoic tracts, sometimes containing air, between the anus or rectum and the perianal surface or vagina. Transperineal ultrasound enables a description of the anatomical relationship of the fistulas with the anal sphincters and can provide a correct classification of perianal fistulas according to the Parks system, with a sensitivity > 85% [28].

Transperineal ultrasound is also useful for the follow-up of perianal fistulas in CD [29]. Rasul and colleagues carried out a study aimed at determining whether the appearance of perianal fistulas at transperineal ultrasound is predictive of a response to infliximab and whether clinical improvement after infliximab is associated with the ultrasonographic closure of fistula tracts. Thirty-five patients with CD and perianal fistulas were assessed by transperineal ultrasound before and up to 48 weeks after infliximab. Transperineal ultrasound identified more fistulas than appreciated clinically, as well as the presence of unsuspected fluid collections. In the short term (8 weeks), approximately half of the patients had complete clinical closure of their fistulas, while transperineal ultrasound showed complete healing in only one in seven. Those with healing at transperineal ultrasound had a much longer time to relapse than those who did not. Baseline fistula characteristics on transperineal ultrasound did not predict either clinical or ultrasonographic healing at the end of the study [29]. Like other studies using transanal ultrasound and MRI, these data confirm that even though fistulas may have clinically healed in the short term with biological therapy, they may still be detectable at transperineal ultrasound such that long-term therapy may be required to completely heal the fistulous tract. Conversely, documentation of complete healing might allow a subset of patients to discontinue infliximab maintenance therapy, with a lower risk of relapse.

References

1. Vermeire S, Van Assche G, Rutgeerts P (2007) Perianal Crohn's disease: Classification and clinical evaluation. Dig Liver Dis 39:959-62
2. Williams DR, Coller JA, Corman ML, et al. (1981) Anal complications in Crohn's disease. Dis Colon Rectum 24:22-4
3. Schwartz DA, Pemberton JH, Sandborn WJ (2001) Diagnosis and treatment of perianal fistulas in Crohn's disease. Ann Intern Med 135:906-10
4. Schwartz D, Loftus EV, Tremaine WJ, et al (2002) The natural history of fistulizing Crohn's disease in Olmsted County, Minnesota. Gastroenterology 122:875-80
5. Present D (2003) Crohn's fistula: current concepts in management. Gastroenterology 124:1629-35
6. Parks A (1976) The pathogenesis and treatment of fistula-in-ano. Br Med J 1:463-9
7. American Gastroenterological Association Medical Position Statement: perianal Crohn's disease (2003). Gastroenterology 125:1503-7
8. Halligan S, Stoker J (2006) Imaging of fistula in ano. Radiology 239:18-33
9. Poen AC, Felt-Bersma RJ, Eijsbouts QA et al. (1998) Hydrogen peroxide-enhanced transanal ultrasound in the assessment of fistula-in-ano. Dis Colon Rectum 41:1147-52
10. Sloots CE, Felt-Bersma RJ, Poen AC et al. (2001) Assessment and classification of fistula-in-ano in patients with Crohn's disease by hydrogen peroxide enhanced transanal ultrasound. Int J Colorectal Dis 16:292-7
11. Schwartz DA, Wiersema MJ, Dudiak KM, et al. (2001) A comparison of endoscopic ultrasound, magnetic resonance imaging, and exam under anesthesia for evaluation of Crohn's perianal fistulas. Gastroenterology 121:1064-72
12. West RL, van der Woude CJ, Hansen BE, et al. (2004) Clinical and endosonographic effect of ciprofloxacin on the treatment of perianal fistulae in Crohn's disease with infliximab: a double-blind placebo-controlled study. Aliment Pharmacol Ther 20:1329-6
13. Caprilli R, Gassull MA, Escher JC, et al. (2006) European Crohn's and Colitis Organisation. European evidence based consensus on the diagnosis and management of Crohn's disease: special situations. Gut 55: 36-58
14. Beets-Tan RG, Beets GL, van der Hoop AG, et al. (2001) Preoperative MR imaging of anal fistulas: does it really help the surgeon? Radiology 218:75-84
15. Van Assche G, Vanbeckevoort D, Bielen D, et al. (2003) Magnetic resonance imag- ing of the effects of infliximab on perianal fistulizing Crohn's disease. Am J Gastroenterol 98:332-9

16. Horsthuis K, Lavini C, Bipat S, et al. (2009) Perianal Crohn dis- ease:evaluation of dynamic contrast-enhanced MR imaging as an indicator of disease activity. Radiology 251:380-7
17. Caprioli F, Losco A, Viganò C, et al. (2006) Computer-assisted evaluation of perianal fistula activity by means of anal ultrasound in patients with Crohn's disease. Am J Gastroenterol 101:1551-8
18. Losco A, Viganò C, Conte D, et al. (2009) Assessing the activity of perianal Crohn's disease: comparison of clinical indices and computer-assisted anal ultrasound. Inflamm Bowel Dis 15:742-9
19. Present DH, Rutgeerts P, Targan S, et al. (1999) Infliximab for the treatment of fistulas in patients with Crohn's disease. N Engl J Med 340:1398-405
20. Spradlin NM, Wise PE, Herline AJ, et al. (2008) A randomized prospective trial of endoscopic ultrasound to guide combination medical and surgical treatment for Crohn's perianal fistulas. Am J Gastroenterol 103:2527-35
21. Ardizzone S, Maconi G, Colombo E, et al. (2004) Perianal fistulae following infliximab treatment: clinical and endosonographic outcome. Inflamm Bowel Dis 10:91-6
22. Schwartz DA, White CM, Wise PE, Herline AJ (2005) Use of endoscopic ultrasound to guide combination medical and surgical therapy for patients with Crohn's perianal fistulas. Inflamm Bowel Dis 11:727-32
23. Giovannini M, Bories E, Moutardier V, et al. (2003) Drainage of deep pelvic abscesses using therapeutic echo endoscopy. Endoscopy 35:511-4
24. Rubens DJ, Strang JG, Bogineni-Misra S, et al. (1998) Transperineal sonography of the rectum: Anatomy and pathology revealed by sonography compared with CT and MR imaging. AJR Am J Roentgenol 170:637-42.7.
25. Stewart LK, McGee J, Wilson SR (2001) Transperineal and transvaginal sonography of perianal inflammatory disease. AJR Am J Roentgenol 177:627-32
26. Wedemeyer J, Kirchhoff T, Sellge G, et al. (2004) Transcutaneous perianal sonography: A sensitive method for the detection of perianal inflammatory lesions in Crohn's disease. World J Gastroenterol 10:2859-63
27. Mallouhi A, Bonatti H, Peer S, et al. (2004) Detection and characterization of perianal inflammatory disease: Accuracy of transperineal combined gray scale and color Doppler sonography. J Ultrasound Med 23:19-27
28. Maconi G, Ardizzone S, Greco S, et al. (2007) Transperineal ultrasound in the detection of perianal and rectovaginal fistulae in Crohn's disease. Am J Gastroenterol 102:2214-9
29. Rasul I, Wlson SR, MacRae H et al. (2003) Clinical and radiological response after Infliximab treatment for perianal fistulizing Crohn's disease. Am J Gastroenterol 99:82-8

Ulcerative Colitis

13

Giovanni Maconi, Federica Furfaro and Cristina Bezzio

13.1 Introduction

Although perianal disease is well recognized as a major complication of Crohn's disease (CD), its association with ulcerative colitis (UC) has been reported in up to 20–25% of patients [1-4]. Anorectal complications in UC patients include conditions such as hemorrhoids, skin tags, anal strictures, fissures, fistulas, and abscesses. Recent studies have focused on fistulas and abscesses, which are major complications of UC after ileal-pouch-anal-anastomosis (IPAA), although the spontaneous occurrence of these lesions has been reported in up to 5% of patients with an initial diagnosis of UC. In approximately 25% of these patients, the findings may change the initial diagnosis of UC over time [4].

Like CD, in UC complicated by perianal fistulas there is a greater and earlier requirement for steroids, immunomodulators and biological therapy, mainly due to the perianal disease itself. The development of perianal fistulas occurs predominantly in UC patients with active disease and in the complex perianal disease in UC patients, whose diagnosis therefore changes to CD or unclassified colitis. Zabana et al. [4] showed that in more than one third of patients with UC and complex perianal disease, the initial diagnosis changed whereas this was not the case in any patient with simple perianal disease. This observation supports the need for an extensive work-up to rule out CD in patients with UC who develop or present with complex perianal disease. This is of relevance considering the risk of surgery and the potential surgical com-

G. Maconi (✉)
Gastroenterology Unit, Department of Biomedical and Clinical Sciences
Luigi Sacco University Hospital
Milan, Italy
e-mail: giovanni.maconi@unimi.it

M.Tonolini and G. Maconi (eds.), *Imaging of Perianal Inflammatory Diseases*,
DOI: 10.1007/978-88-470-2847-0_13, © Springer-Verlag Italia 2013

plications experienced by UC patients who need proctocolectomy with IPAA to treat the UC. In fact, the prevalence of colectomy in UC patients with perianal disease is nearly double that of patients without [4]. In addition, clinical signs favoring the diagnosis of CD in UC patients, such as the presence of perianal disease, are risk factors for the development of pouch-related fistulas [5, 6]. In turn, fistulizing disease after IPAA is associated with a high failure/stoma rate (approximately 46%) despite treatment with infliximab and/or immunosuppressants. These observations strongly highlight the importance of an accurate diagnosis of fistulas in every patient with UC as well as accurate re-assessment of the intestinal disease.

Considering that the highest accuracy in the diagnosis and classification of perianal fistulas is usually reached with the use of more than one imaging technique, transanal or perineal ultrasound could be added to magnetic resonance imaging for this purpose. Moreover, besides the assessment of perianal complications, transanal and perineal ultrasound can be used to examine the wall of the rectum in order to evaluate disease activity and the function of the pouch-anal anastomosis in patients with incontinence or obstructed defecation.

13.2 Transanal Ultrasound

Transanal ultrasound can accurately assess and classify perianal complications of UC such as fistulas and abscesses, whether spontaneously occurring or complicating IPAA. Moreover, sonographic assessment of the rectal wall also has been proposed as a diagnostic tool to differentiate UC from CD, to assess the severity of disease and for prognostic purposes.

The fistula tracts and abscesses complicating UC resemble those of Crohn's disease. Fistulous tracts may be identified as hypoechoic, round to oval structures in an intersphincteric location, sometimes with internal hyperechoic echoes as a result of gas or air within an abscess or a fistulous tract. An opening within the mucosa of the anal canal or within the rectum may present as a gap or disruption of the integrity of the echostructure of the normal wall (Fig. 13.1).

The fistulas in UC may be difficult to assess, especially in patients with IPAA, in whom the diagnosis and classification of these lesions are hampered by deformation of the pouch-anal anastomosis, defects of the anal sphincters, and the presence of sinuses and folds that may simulate the presence of incomplete perianal fistulas. However, to date, no study has assessed the accuracy of transanal ultrasound in detecting fistulas and abscesses in patients with IPAA.

Transanal ultrasound may reveal defects in the anal sphincters and assess wall and peri-pouch changes. A study that quantified the anatomical changes of the anal sphincters after IPAA correlated these findings with anal manometry and fecal incontinence in 23 patients [9]. The results showed that IPAA leads to a reduction in the thickness of the internal anal sphincter (mean 1.16 mm), with tapering or gaps probably caused by direct trauma to the sphincter because of

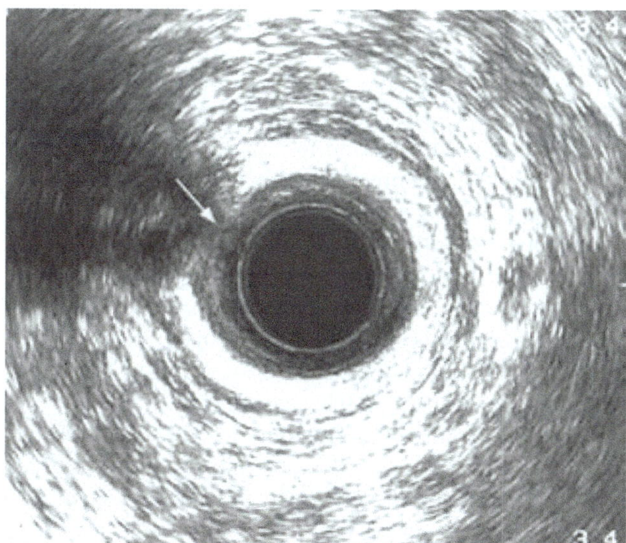

Fig. 13.1 Perianal fistula in a 39-year-old man with ulcerative colitis. Note the hypoechoic area and disruption of the normal wall structure at the site of the internal opening

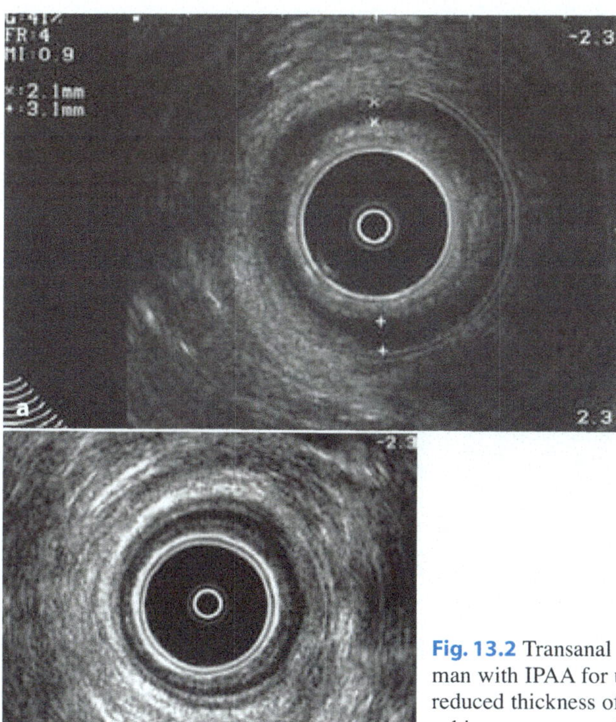

Fig. 13.2 Transanal ultrasound in a 42-year-old man with IPAA for ulcerative colitis. **a** Note the reduced thickness of the internal and external sphincters compared with **b** that of the normal anal canal in an age-comparable male patient with ulcerative colitis

mucosectomy and/or denervation (Fig. 13.2); however, the reduction in the internal anal sphincter thickness did not correlate with continence. In patients with pouchitis, transanal ultrasound may show a variably increased wall thickening, hypertrophy of the peri-pouch fat, and enlarged lymphnodes (Fig. 13.3).

With the high resolution of transanal ultrasound in imaging the rectal walls and assessing the depth of intestinal inflammation, this technique has been proposed to differentiate UC from CD and infectious colitis, to assess disease activity, and to predict the response to medical treatment and the need for surgery, both in patients with active UC and in those with IPAA.

Preliminary results showed that in UC, rectal wall thickness as assessed by intraluminal sonography using transanal or miniaturized probes in combination with endoscopy correlates with disease activity and may predict both the response to medical therapy and the occurrence of relapse [10, 11].

Furthermore, since CD tends to be transmural while UC is a superficial mucosal inflammatory process, hopes were raised that trans-rectal ultrasound would be effective in discriminating cases of otherwise indeterminate colitis. However, such efforts have been largely disappointing [12], although a recent pilot study showed that transrectal ultrasound elastography may be a promising diagnostic tool to differentiate UC from CD. Specifically, the stiffness of the bowel wall, as assessed according to the strain ratio, was shown to better differentiate inflammatory bowel disease than a simple measurement of rectal wall thickness [13], while in a small study the detection of perirectal lymph nodes in patients with nonspecific or suspected infectious colitis was shown to suggest a diagnosis of associated UC or to predict the development of a chronic colitis [14].

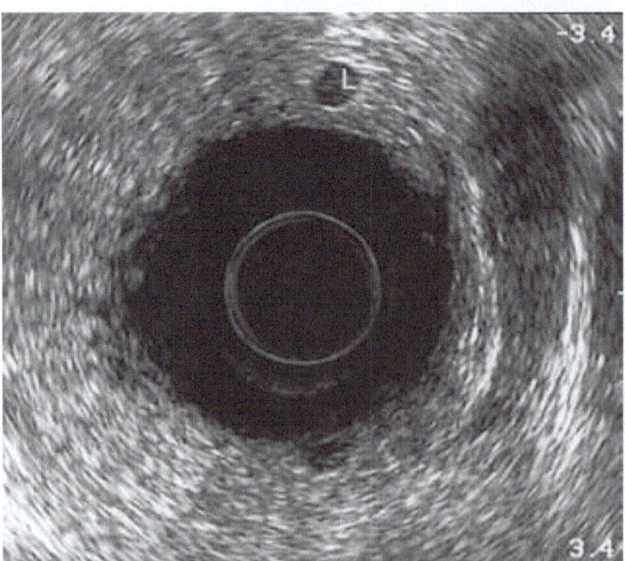

Fig. 13.3 A 34-year-old man with pouchitis. Transanal ultrasound shows increased wall thickening, hypertrophy of the peri-pouch fat, and enlarged lymph-nodes

13.3 Trans-perineal Ultrasound

Perineal ultrasound can be used to assess the wall of the distal rectum and anorectal junction in the setting of an assessment of a perianal fistula and the function of the pouch-anal anastomosis in patients with IPAA in whom obstructed defecation and fecal incontinence have developed.

Perineal ultrasound, performed using high-frequency curved microconvex and linear-array probes, assesses fistulous and sinus tracts as well as abscesses and collections, documenting their relationship with the anal canal, the scrotum in men, and the labia and vagina in women. In particular, perineal ultrasound is useful to detect perianal fistulas and inflammatory tissue or masses located outside the field of view of transanal ultrasound, or when the latter exam cannot be performed in a patient with severe anal pain or stricture (Figs. 13.4 and 13.5). Perineal ultrasound can also be employed to differentiate superficial lesions that simulate perianal fistula, such as pilonidal sinus. The latter originates subcutaneously, most likely from a chronic infection of a hair follicle.

In patients with IPAA, perianal ultrasound may be a valid screening method to assess inflammatory complications and, when used in real-time dynamic assessment, also a practical tool to assess the function of IPAA in patients with symptoms suggesting mechanical or functional complications, such as evacuation disorders or obstructed defecation.

Pouchitis is the most common inflammatory complication of IPAA, occurring in up to 46% of patients. It is an idiopathic inflammatory disease of the ileal reservoir that is a form of recurrent inflammatory bowel disease. On ultrasound, pouchitis may show subtle wall thickening in the pouch and a large volume of fluid feces within its lumen. This complication may occur in patients with anal hypertonus or in those with stenosis of the anal canal such that transanal ultrasound may be painful and difficult to perform.

The functional outcome of IPAA depends to a large extent on the postoperative function of both sphincters, which can be well studied using transanal and transperineal ultrasound. In particular, transperineal ultrasound offers an alternative imaging modality to describe the integrity of the anal sphincter complexes and to document changes in their volume, length, and average thickness [15, 16]. Dynamic perineal ultrasound enables examination of the perineum and the pelvis both at rest and on straining in patients with fecal incontinence, evacuatory difficult and obstructed defecation [17-19], and thus providing useful information. It can also assess the function of a pouch-anal anastomosis.

The assessment of specific ultrasound parameters, such as (a) the length of the anus and its shortening during squeezing, (b) the distance between the posterior margin of the ano-pouch junction and the pubis (corresponding to the length of the puborectalis muscle), (c) the ano-pouch angle, and (d) the distance between this point and the axis passing through the central portion of the pubis during straining and squeezing, can provide valuable information in patients with IPAA dysfunction (Fig. 13.6).

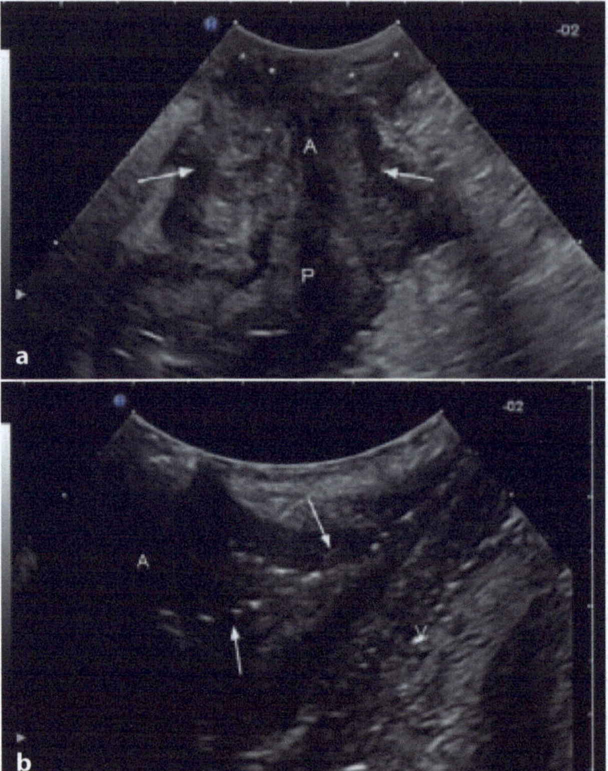

Fig. 13.4 A 25-year-old woman with peripouch inflammatory tissue and pouch fistulas. **a** Longitudinal perianal ultrasound section, showing peripouch superficial (*asterisks*) and deep (*arrows*) inflammatory hypoechoic tissue. **b** Coronal perianal ultrasound section in the same patients, showing fistulous tracts (*arrows*) and inflammatory tissue extended to vagina (*V*). *P* pouch, *A* pouch-anal anastomosis

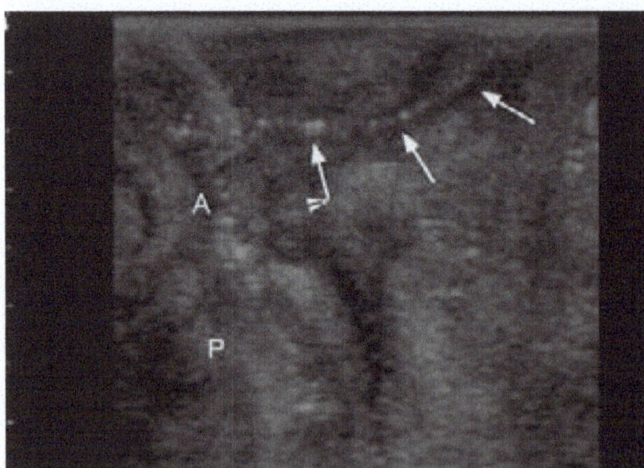

Fig. 13.5 A 20-year-old woman, with anastomotic stricture and suspected pouch-vaginal fistula. Transperineal ultrasound revealed a hypoechoic tract with gaseous content (*arrows*), suggesting a fistulous tract, between the pouch-anal anatomosis and distal tract of the vagina. *P* pouch, *A* pouch anal anastomosis

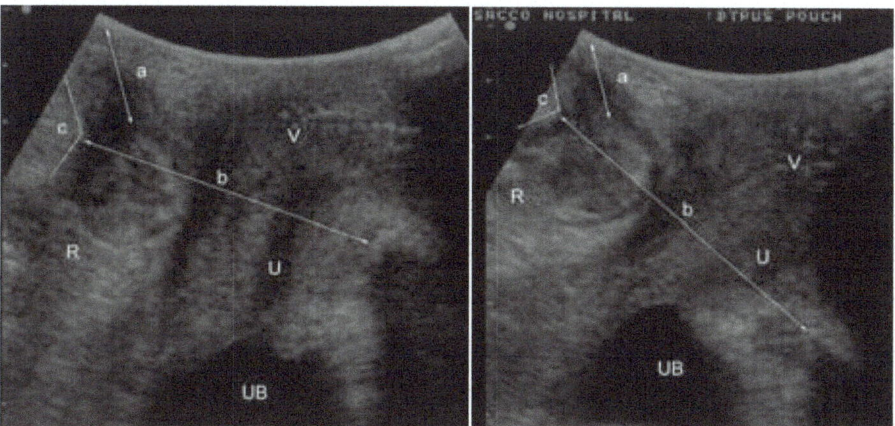

Fig. 13.6 Parameters commonly used to assess to IPAA function at rest (*left panel*) and on squeezing (*right panel*). *a* Length of the anus; *b* distance between the posterior margin of the ano-pouch junction and the pubis; *c* ano-pouch angle. *UB* urinary bladder, *R* rectum, *V* vagina, *U* urethra

References

1. de Dombal F, Watts J, Watkinson G, Goligher J (1996) Incidence and management of anorectal abscess, fistula, and fissure in patients with ulcerative colitis. Dis Colon Rectum 9:201-16
2. Edwards F, Truelove SC (1964) The course and prognosis of ulcerative colitis. Part III Complications. Gut 32:1-22
3. Fuzy PZ (1961) Surgical management of anorectal complications of chronic ulcerative colitis. South Med J 54:795-817
4. Zabana Y, Van Domselaar M, Garcia-Planella E et al (2011) Perianal disease in patients with ulcerative colitis: A case-control study. J Crohn's Colitis 5:338-341
5. Melton GB, Kiran RP, Fazio VW, et al (2010) Do preoperative factors predict subsequent diagnosis of Crohn's disease after ileal pouch-anal anastomosis for ulcerative or indeterminate colitis? Colorectal Dis 12:1026-32
6. Tekkis PP, Fazio VW, Remzi F, et al (2005) Risk factors associated with ileal pouch-related fistula following restorative proctocolectomy. Br J Surg 92:1270-6
7. Haveran LA, Sehgal R, Poritz LS, et al (2011) Infliximab and/or azathioprine in the treatment of Crohn's disease-like complications after IPAA. Dis Colon Rectum 54:15-20
8. Nisar PJ, Kiran RP, Shen B, et al (2011) Factors associated with ileoanal pouch failure in patients developing early or late pouch-related fistula. Dis Colon Rectum. 54:446-53
9. Silvis R, van Eekelen JW, Delemarre JB, Gooszen HG (1995) Endosonography of the anal sphincter after ileal pouch-anal anastomosis. Relation with anal manometry and fecal continence.Dis Colon Rectum 38:383-8
10. Yoshizawa S, Kobayashi K, Katsumata T, et al (2007) Clinical usefulness of EUS for active ulcerative colitis. Gastrointest Endosc 65:253-60
11. Higaki S, Nohara H, Saitoh Y, et al (2002) Increased rectal wall thickness may predict relapse in ulcerative colitis: a pilot follow-up study by ultrasonographic colonoscopy. Endoscopy 34:212-9
12. Lew RJ, Ginsberg GG (2002) The role of endoscopic ultrasound in inflammatory bowel disease. Gastrointest Endosc Clin N Am 12:561-71

13. Rustemovic N, Cukovic-Cavka S, Brinar M, et al (2011) A pilot study of transrectal endoscopic ultrasound elastography in inflammatory bowel disease. BMC Gastroenterol 11:113
14. Gast P (1999) Endorectal ultrasound in infectious colitis may predict development of chronic colitis. Endoscopy 31:265-8
15. Peschers UM, DeLancey JO, Schaer GN, Schuessler B (2007) Exoanal ultrasound of the anal sphincter: normal anatomy and sphincter defects. Br J Obstet Gynaecol 104:999-1003
16. Gosselink MP, West RL, Kuipers EJ, et al (2005) Integrity of the anal sphincters after pouch-anal anastomosis: evaluation with three-dimensional endoanal ultrasonography. Dis Colon Rectum 48:1728-1735
17. Beer-Gabel M, Assoulin Y, Amitai M, Bardan E (2008) A comparison of dynamic transperineal ultrasound (DTP-US. with dynamic evacuation proctography (DEP) in the diagnosis of cul de sac hernia (enterocele) in patients with evacuatory dysfunction. Int J Colorectal Dis 23:513-9
18. Martellucci J, Naldini G (2011) Clinical relevance of transperineal ultrasound compared with evacuation proctography for the evaluation of patients with obstructed defaecation. Colorectal Dis 13:1167-72
19. Zbar A (2010) Dynamic magnetic resonance imaging and transperineal sonography in the assessment of patients presenting primarily with evacuatory difficulty: a short position paper. Acta Chir Iugosl 57:97-104

Cryptoglandular Fistulas

14

Giovanni Maconi, Giulio A. Santoro and Cristina Bezzio

14.1 Introduction

Cryptoglandular anal fistulas arise from inflammation of the proctodeal glands of the intersphincteric space. The mucus secretions of the anal glands empty into the anal crypts, thereby lubricating the anus. Anal glands are present in the subepithelium and the internal sphincter, with a large number also deeply sited within the intersphincteric space [1]. Infection of these intersphincteric glands is thought to give rise to an intersphincteric abscess if the draining duct is blocked by the resulting infectious debris. The abscess may resolve by spontaneous drainage into the anal canal or it may progress to an acute anorectal abscess that, in most cases, subsequently develops into a perianal fistula. Perianal fistula is therefore a communication between an opening at the level of the dentate line and in the perianal region represents the chronic manifestation of the intersphincteric abscess.

In most cases, the internal opening of cryptoglandular fistulas is at the 6 o'clock position, since the anal glands are more abundant posteriorly. In such cases, the anatomic course by which the fistula reaches the perianal skin may vary, with some routes being linear while others are tortuous, penetrating, and involving the muscles of the anal sphincter and surrounding tissues.

In an early study by Morgan and Thompson (1956) it was postulated that intersphincteric abscesses follow the septal fibers of the terminal fibroelastic, conjoint longitudinal tendon traversing the external sphincter and ending at the ischiorectal fossa [2]. This proposal was investigated by Parks et al. (1976), who examined 400 consecutive patients referred to the surgeons at St Mark's

G. Maconi (✉)
Gastroenterology Unit, Department of Biomedical and Clinical Sciences
Luigi Sacco University Hospital
Milan, Italy
e-mail: giovanni.maconi@unimi.it

M.Tonolini and G. Maconi (eds.), *Imaging of Perianal Inflammatory Diseases*,
DOI: 10.1007/978-88-470-2847-0_14, © Springer-Verlag Italia 2013

Hospital in London. Based on the collected data, perianal fistulas were classified into four groups with respect to their route and their relation to the internal and external anal sphincters: intersphincteric, transsphincteric, suprasphincteric, and extrasphincteric [3]. It should be noted that the series of Parks et al. was inevitably influenced by the specialized nature of St Mark's Hospital, where most patients were either operated on or otherwise admitted for the treatment of Crohn's disease, a bias acknowledged by Parks himself. Thus, Parks et al. did not describe superficial or submucosal fistulas in their series such that their results do not concur with those of other wide series in which only patients with never operated on cryptoglandular fistulas were included; in these cases, neither suprasphincteric nor extrasphincteric fistulas were found [4].

Most fistulas arise as a single primary tract, whereas recurrent fistulas may develop ramifications and therefore extend away from the original tract. In fact, Sloots et al. (2001), using hydrogen peroxide enhanced transanal ultrasound, showed that all never operated on cryptoglandular fistulas-in-ano were intersphincteric or transsphincteric whilst recurrent fistulas were suprasphincteric or extrasphincteric in 15% and ramified in 27% [5].

The extensions in recurrent cryptoglandular fistulas, as with those in Crohn's disease, may be intersphincteric, ischioanal, and pararectal or supralevator. The morphology of these extensions may suggest fistulous tracts or abscesses. The ischioanal fossa is the most common site for the extensions but intersphincteric extension along the horizontal plane, also known as a "horseshoe fistula," is frequent as well.

14.2 Transanal Ultrasound

Transanal ultrasound has been extensively used for the classification of fistula-in-ano. It is simple, rapid, and well tolerated by most patients. Due to its ability to provide images of the anal sphincter complex with very high spatial resolution, it is considered the method of choice for identifying small intersphincteric abscesses that are difficult to resolve using other imaging techniques and for assessing the internal opening of a perianal fistulas, which is usually positioned directly at the probe surface [6]. However, it should be considered that tracts extending up to the anal mucosal surface may be missed. The internal opening is usually revealed as a hypoechoic focus in the intersphincteric space that abuts the internal sphincter, often with a small corresponding defect in the internal sphincter (Fig. 14.1). Due to their linear route, intersphincteric fistulas are usually very well visualized at anal endosonography. Transsphincteric fistulas are seen as hypoechoic tracts that cross the external sphincter to reach the ischioanal fossa (Fig. 14.2). Extensions of these fistulas are often identified as hypoechoic fluid collections. Nonetheless, while an intersphincteric horseshoe extension may be well imaged by transverse endosonogram (Fig 14.3), ischioanal or supralevator extensions may be

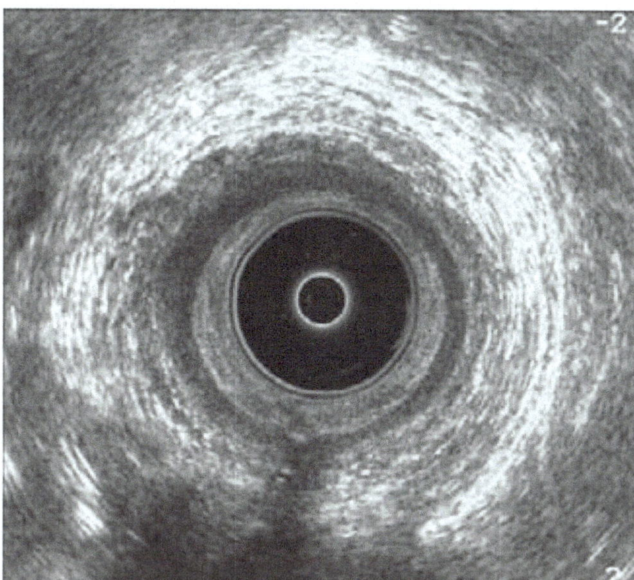

Fig. 14.1 Transanal ultrasound showing an internal opening of a transsphincteric fistula, seen as a hypoechoic focus in the intersphincteric space that abuts the internal sphincter, with a small corresponding defect in the internal sphincter

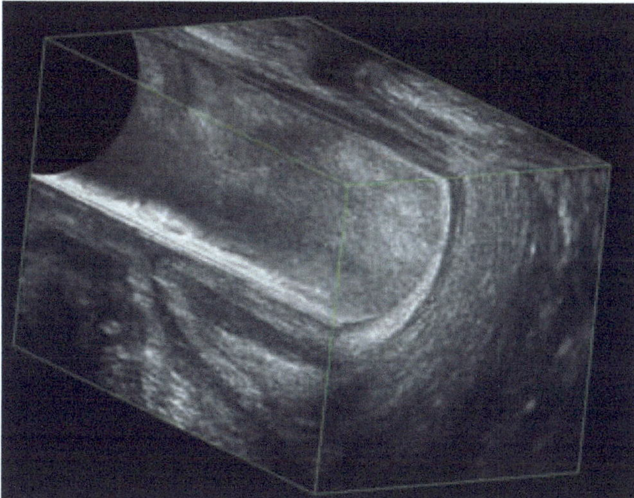

Fig. 14.2 On transanal ultrasound, transsphincteric fistulas are seen as hypoechoic tracts that cross the external sphincter to reach the ischioanal fossa

missed or incompletely imaged due to insufficient penetration of the ultrasound beam beyond the external sphincter. Accordingly, transanal ultrasound is also disadvantaged by its inability to image the surgically important coronal plane, making it potentially very difficult to distinguish supralevator from infralevator extensions.

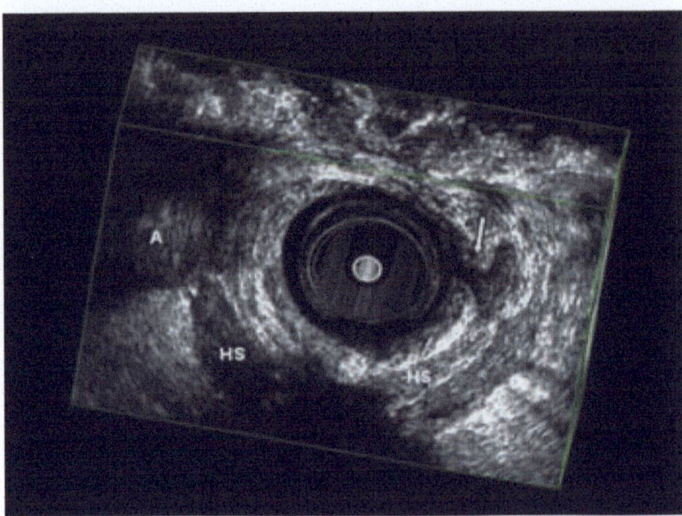

Fig. 14.3 Transanal ultrasound showing an intersphincteric horseshoe extension of a transsphincteric fistula (*arrow*). *A* Abscess, *HS* horseshoe extension

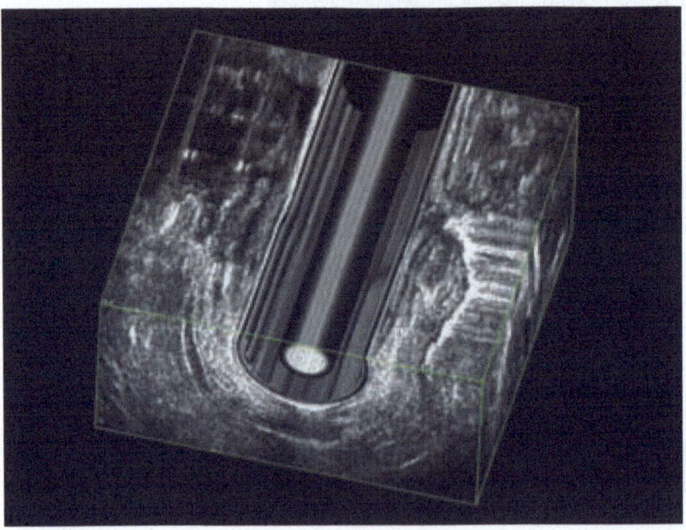

Fig. 14.4 Three-dimensional transrectal ultrasound coupled with the injection of hydrogen peroxide into the external opening of the fistula, showing a complex fistula with extension

To overcome this disadvantage, 3D acquisition, possibly coupled with the injection of hydrogen peroxide into the external opening of the fistula, has become widely adopted (Fig. 14.4) [7]. In 21 patients with a cryptoglandular

Table 14.1 Agreement ratios and k values of 3D hydrogen-peroxide-enhanced ultrasound (HPUS), endoanal magnetic resonance imaging (MRI), and surgery for the classification of perianal fistulas [8]

	3D HPUS and surgery	Endoanal MRI and surgery	3D HPUS and endoanal MRI
Primary tract	81%	90% k = 0.47	90%
Circular secondary tract	67%	57% k = 0.07	71% k = 0.45
Linear secondary tract	76%	81%	95%
Internal opening site	86% k = 0.67	86% k = 0.69	90% k = 0.82

fistula, West et al. (2003) compared 3D-hydrogen peroxide-enhanced transanal ultrasound with endoanal MRI and surgery. Agreement regarding the classification of the primary fistula tract was 81% for hydrogen-peroxide-enhanced 3D-transanal ultrasound and surgery, 90% for endoanal MRI and surgery, and 90% for hydrogen-peroxide-enhanced 3D transanal ultrasound and endoanal MRI. For secondary tracts, agreement was 67%, 57%, and 71%, respectively, in case of circular tracts and 76%, 81 %, and 71%, respectively, in case of linear tracts. Agreement for the location of an internal opening was 86% for hydrogen-peroxide-enhanced 3D transanal ultrasound and surgery, 86% for endoanal MRI and surgery, and 90% for hydrogen-peroxide-enhanced 3D transanal ultrasound and endoanal MRI (Table 14.1) [8].

Besides its use in the classification of perianal fistulas and the detection of extensions and complications, transanal ultrasound might be valuable in defining the nature of the fistula, as the fistulas occurring in Crohn's disease have a markedly different appearance and course than those that develop in the non-Crohn's population [9]. However, some fistulas in Crohn's patients are successfully treated with means designed for cryptoglandular fistulas. To distinguish the anal fistulas of Crohn's disease from cryptoglandular fistulas that occur in patients with this disease, Blom et al. (2011) suggested that three endoanal ultrasonographic criteria be taken into account: (1) bifurcation or secondary extension, (2) cross-sectional width ≥ 3 mm, and (3) the content of the hyperechoic secretions. The presence of one or none of these criteria identifies cryptoglandular fistulas while if two or three criteria are confirmed then the diagnosis is most likely Crohn's fistula, characterized by longer duration, greater number of previous operations, and a higher perianal Crohn's disease activity index [10]. Also, the anatomical distribution of fistula subtypes among Crohn's and non-Crohn's fistula differs significantly since fistulas with a posterior external opening are more frequently of the cryptogenic type [9].

References

1. McColl I (1967) Comparative anatomy and pathology of anal glands. Ann R Coll Surg Engl 40:36-6
2. Morgan CN, Thompson HR (1956) Surgical anatomy of the anal canal with special reference to the surgical importance of the internal sphincter and conjoint longitudinal muscle. Ann Coll Surg Engl 19: 88
3. Parks AG, Gordon PH, Hardcastle JD (1976) A classification of fistula-in-ano. Br J Surg 63:1-12
4. Eisenhammer S (1978) The final evaluation and classifcation of the surgical treatment of the primary anorectal cryptoglandular intermuscular (intersphinteric) fistulous abcess and fistula. Dis Colon Rectum 21: 237-54.
5. Sloots CE, Felt-Bersma RJ, Poen AC, Cuesta MA (2001) Assessment and classification of never operated and recurrent cryptoglandular fistulas-in-ano using hydrogen peroxide enhanced transanal ultrasound. Colorectal Dis 3:422-6
6. Buchanan GN, Halligan S, Bartram CI, et al. (2004) Clinical examination, endosonography, and MR imaging in preoperative assessment of fistula in ano: comparison with outcome-based reference standard. Radiology 233:674-81
7. Santoro GA, Fortling B (2007) The advantages of volume rendering in three-dimensional endosonography of the anorectum. Dis Colon Rectum 50:359-68
8. West RL, Zimmerman DD, Dwarkasing S, et al. (2003) Prospective comparison of hydrogen peroxide-enhanced three-dimensional endoanal ultrasonography and endoanal magnetic resonance imaging of perianal fistulas. Dis Colon Rectum 46:1407–1415
9. Coremans G, Dockx S, Wyndaele J, Hendrickx A (2003) Do anal fistulas in Crohn's disease behave differently and defy Goodsall's rule more frequently than fistulas that are cryptoglandular in origin? Am J Gastroenterol 98:2732-5
10. Blom J, Nyström PO, Gunnarsson U, Strigård K (2011) Endoanal ultrasonography may distinguish Crohn's anal fistulae from cryptoglandular fistulae in patients with Crohn's disease: a cross-sectional study. Tech Coloproctol 15:327-30

Cancer in Perianal Fistulas 15

Giovanni Maconi, Federica Furfaro and Cristina Bezzio

15.1 Introduction

The development of cancer at the site of a chronic fistula in the absence of Crohn's disease (CD) is very rare. However, also in long-standing CD complicated by chronic sinuses or fistulas, the occurrence of carcinoma related to the fistula is seldom, with an incidence of less than 0.7% of CD patients [1]. A review of 40 cases of anorectal carcinomas in patients with fistulizing CD showed that only in 22 (55%) patients could a definite association with an anorectal fistula be established. These cancers were classified as squamous cell carcinomas (10), adenocarcinomas (11), and basaloid carcinoma (1) [1]. The tumors presented several years (range 14–20 years) after the initial diagnosis of CD [1, 2]. Although the causative relationship between CD and the carcinomatous transformation of anorectal fistulas is not fully understood, it has been suggested that delayed wound healing, constant mucosal regeneration and high cell turnover rates, and the immunosuppressive therapies used to treat CD all play a role [3, 4].

Cancer in a perianal fistula is very difficult to diagnose. In particular, it is difficult to establish whether the carcinoma has developed in a chronic fistula or whether the fistula is the result of the cancer's expansion. The lesion may be initially mistaken for an abscess or mass within the fistula tract. Moreover, the diagnosed is often delayed since routine proctological examination may be limited by pain, strictures, embarrassment, and lack of patient cooperation. In addition, conventional diagnostic imaging techniques (e.g., MRI or transanal ultrasound) may provide inconclusive results. Examination under anesthesia

G. Maconi (✉)
Gastroenterology Unit, Department of Biomedical and Clinical Sciences
Luigi Sacco University Hospital
Milan, Italy
e-mail: giovanni.maconi@unimi.it

M.Tonolini and G. Maconi (eds.), *Imaging of Perianal Inflammatory Diseases*,
DOI: 10.1007/978-88-470-2847-0_15, © Springer-Verlag Italia 2013

may also fail to achieve the diagnosis if a biopsy or a curettage of the fistulous tract is not performed [1, 2]. Biopsies or curettage of the fistula should be obtained in patients who complain of increased pain or discharge or bleeding as well as in patients with an increase in the size of the fistulous tract or in whom perianal lymph nodes are detected. Unfortunately, however, in most patients the tumor is in an advanced stage at the time of its detection, with a poor prognosis. In fact, at the time of presentation, the tumors are over 5 cm in diameter in 80% of the cases and generally associated with metastasis to the inguinal and retrorectal lymph nodes [5-7]. Therefore, a high degree of suspicion for malignancy is the key to an early diagnosis and thus to early treatment [6].

15.2 Imaging Features

Transanal ultrasound, CT scan, and MRI, although not diagnostic, can increase the degree of suspicion of cancer and are fundamental in evaluating disease extension.

In patients with recurrent chronic perianal fistulas characterized by changes in fistula-associated clinical features, such as bleeding, increased perianal pain, or drainage of a more mucoid character, and by changes in the morphological features of the fistula tracts on diagnostic imaging, the possibility of malignancy must be excluded.

In this setting, transanal and transperineal ultrasound may reveal an enlargement of the fistulous tract (which may be hypoechoic and well vascularized on color power Doppler examination), the development of a hypoechoic perianal mass, and frank liquid collections within the fistula wall (especially in cases of mucinous adenocarcinoma). In advanced stages, the presence of perianal lymph nodes may be observed (Fig. 15.1) [8-11].

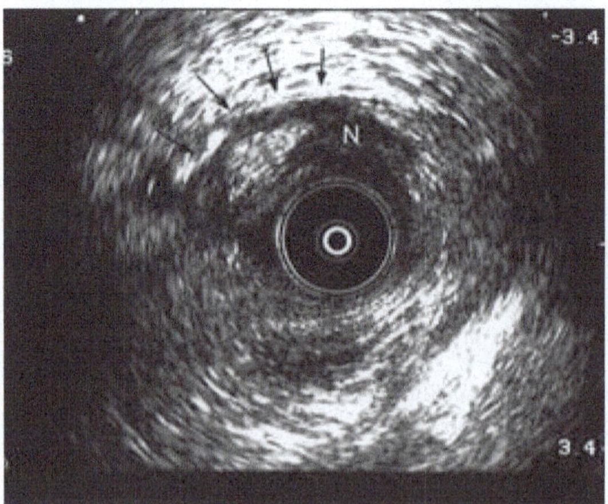

Fig. 15.1 Transanal ultrasonographic appearance of an internal rectal fistula (*arrows*) arising from an ileal cancer and abutting the wall of the distal rectum (*N*). The presence of neoplastic tissue within the fistuolous tract was not detectable with conventional diagnostic methods and was discovered only after surgery, proctectmy, and fistulectomy

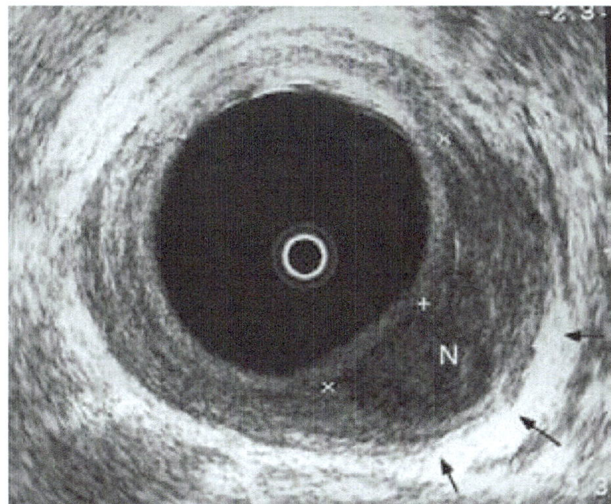

Fig. 15.2 Tumor (N) of the anal canal involving the subepithelium and internal sphincter. The neoplasia is confined to the internal sphincter (*arrows*), leaving intact the external anal sphincter (stage: T2, N0)

Table 15.1 Ultrasound staging of anal malignancy

Stage	Definition
T1	Confined to the subepithelium
T2	Limited to the sphincter muscles
T3	Penetrating the external anal sphincter
T4	Involving adjacent structures

In patients with anorectal cancer presenting with a perianal fistula, imaging diagnosis may be problematic. In this case, transanal ultrasound can be requested to evaluate a palpable mass within the anal canal associated with a perianal fistula. Transanal ultrasound may provide information regarding tumor size, location, depth of the cancer's mural penetration, and of the tumor extension beyond the anal canal through the perineum and into adjacent structures (Fig. 15.2).

Squamous cell carcinomas of the anal canal are rare but require careful staging to select appropriate treatment, typically with combined chemotherapy and radiotherapy. Transanal ultrasound allows tumor staging based on depth of tumor invasion (Table 15.1), which is useful in determining the response to radiotherapy [12] and in monitoring the patient for local recurrence.

References

1. Ky A, Sohn N, Weinstein MA, et al (1998) Carcinoma arising in anorectal fistulas of Crohn's disease. Dis Colon Rectum 41:992-996
2. Ekbom A, Helmick C, Zack M, Adami HO (1990) Increased risk of large-bowel cancer in Crohn's disease with colonic involvement. Lancet 336:357-359
3. Buchman AL, Ament ME, Doty J (1991) Development of squamous cell carcinoma in chronic perineal sinus and wounds in Crohn's disease. Am J Gastroenterol 86:1829-1832
4. Slater G, Greenstein A, Aufses AH Jr (1984) Anal carcinoma in patients with Crohn's disease. Ann Surg 199:348-350
5. Erhan Y, Sakarya A, Aydede H, et al (2003) A case of large mucinous adenocarcinoma arising in a long-standing fistula in ano. Dig Surg 20:69-71
6. Marti L, Nussbaumer P, Breitbach T, Hollinger A (2001) Perianal mucinous adenocarcinoma. A further reason for histological study of anal fistula or anorectal abscess. Chirurg 72:573-577
7. Iesalnieks I, Gaertner WB, Glass H, et al (2010) Fistula-associated anal adenocarcinoma in Crohn's disease. Inflamm Bowel Dis 6:1643-8
8. Navarra G, Ascanelli S, Turini A,, et al (1999) Mucinous adenocarcinoma in chronic anorectal fistula. Chir Ital 51:413-416
9. Getz SB, Ough YD, Patterson RB, et al (1981) Mucinous adenocarcinoma developing in chronic anal fistula: report of two cases and review of the literature. Dis Colon Rectum 24:562
10. Onerheim RM (1988) A case of perianal mucinous adenocarcinoma arising in a fistula-in-ano. A clue to the early pathologic diagnosis. Am J Clin Pathol 89:809-12
11. Jones EA, Morson BC (1984) Mucinous adenocarcinoma in anorectal fistulae. Histopathology 8:279-292
12. Goldman S, Norming U, Svensson C et al (1991) Transanorectal ultrasonography in the staging of anal epidermoid carcinoma. Int J Colorect 6:152-157

Rare Diseases

16

Giovanni Maconi, Elena Bolzacchini and Cristina Bezzio

16.1 Cryptitis

Cryptitis is the localized infection of the anal glands. This unusual condition is identified anoscopically as a pearl of pus beading up from the crypt at the level of the dentate line. The condition may be encountered also in infants due to androgen excess during the fetal stage. The high levels of hormone cause the abnormal development of the crypts of Morgagni, which encourages cryptitis and abscess formation. In most cases, cryptitis and perianal abscess may progress to form a fistula.

Transanal or transperineal ultrasound reveals a small, single, hypo- or anechoic lesion localized at level of the dentate line, at the site of the anal glands. The lesions are usually painful, such that transanal ultrasound is often not possible. In such cases, perineal ultrasound may be preferable, especially in pediatric patients (Fig 16.1).

Treatment relies on local hygiene and systemic antibiotics. However, while in the pediatric population this approach, even without surgical drainage, can minimize the formation of fistula-in-ano, in adults surgical revision may be required to avoid fistula formation [1, 2].

16.2 Perianal Hidradenitis Suppurativa

Hidradenitis suppurativa is a chronic skin disorder affecting areas rich in apocrine glands. It is characterized by the occurrence of boils in the affected sites

G. Maconi (✉)
Gastroenterology Unit, Department of Biomedical and Clinical Sciences
Luigi Sacco University Hospital
Milan, Italy
e-mail: giovanni.maconi@unimi.it

M.Tonolini and G. Maconi (eds.), *Imaging of Perianal Inflammatory Diseases*,
DOI: 10.1007/978-88-470-2847-0_16, © Springer-Verlag Italia 2013

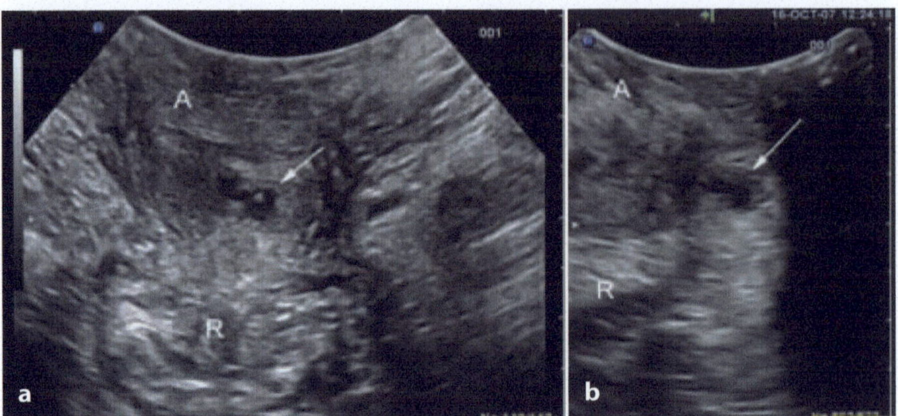

Fig. 16.1 Coronal (**a**) and sagittal (**b**) trans-perineal scans performed in a 36-year old patient with severe perianal pain show a small abscess of the crypt at the level of the dentate line (*arrows*). The symptoms and the lesion disappeared following systemic antibiotic treatment

that gradually enlarge and rupture, with heavy purulence. Hidradenitis suppurativa has a point prevalence of up to 4.1% and is more common in females.

The pathogenesis of this disease is unknown, although genetic factors, hormones, and infection have been implicated. An association with Crohn's disease and arthropathy has also been reported [3, 4].

The perineum is one of the most frequently affected sites, along with the axilla and groin, due to the high density of follicular structures in this area. Disease onset is insidious. Initially, individuals may experience slight discomfort or pruritus in the affected area. Subsequently, a tender papule or deep-seeded nodule develops. While this nodule may slowly resolve, it often expands and coalesces with surrounding nodules to form large, painful inflammatory abscesses that may rupture spontaneously, yielding a purulent discharge. The lesion then heals with fibrosis, dermal contractures, and rope-like elevation of the skin, and double-ended comedones. Sinus tracts may also develop.

Therapy of hidradenitis suppurativa consists primarily of systemic antibiotics and topical antiseptics. Surgical removal of all involved tissue, beyond the clinically involved margins, is the most effective treatment strategy. However, postoperative recurrences are not uncommon. In such cases, ultrasonography can be useful in surgical planning. Ultrasound, performed with high-resolution 7- to 12-MHz linear transducers coupled with color Doppler, reveals hypoechoic areas reflecting edema and inflamed tissue not only of the skin but also of the subcutaneous tissue (Fig. 16.2). Vascularity and a resistance index (RI) typically > 0.40 characterize severe lesions. Usually, these changes are more widespread than expected from clinical examination and the changes visible on ultrasound always extend beyond the clinically identified borders of the lesions [5, 6].

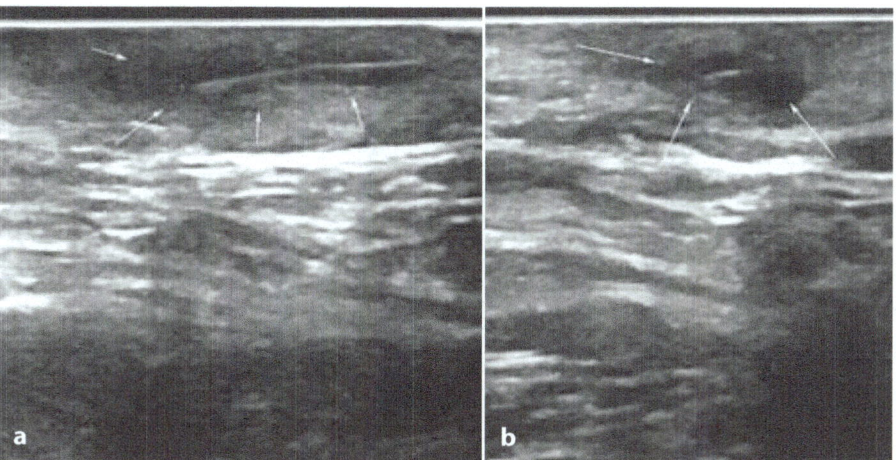

Fig. 16.2 Longitudinal (**a**) and transversal (**b**) scan of a circumscribed hypoechoic and vascularized lesion in the dermal layer (*arrows*), reflecting edema and inflamed tissue in a 32-year-old woman with recurrent perianal hidradenitis suppurativa

16.3 Anal Tuberculosis

Anoperineal tuberculosis (TB) is an exceedingly rare extrapulmonary form of the disease (1% of digestive tract incidence) that must be recognized because it requires specific treatment. Anoperineal TB is most common in men (77–100% of cases) and occurs secondary to a primary site in the lungs. Anal contamination is usually caused by the swallowing of respiratory secretions that contain a large quantity of Koch's bacillus. A pre-existing anal lesion (fissure, erosion, fistula, pilonidal sinus, or scar) is often found [7].

Anoperineal TB should be suspected on the basis of the following criteria: recurring anal fistula or abscess, pulmonary TB, or the presence of an epithelioid granuloma on histologic examination of the excised tissue in the absence of known Crohn's disease (the presence of a giant cell granuloma with caseous necrosis is considered pathognomonic of TB).

Anal TB has a distinct clinical presentation. The ulcerated form typically presents as a superficial ulceration, not hardened, with a hemorrhagic necrotic base that is granular and covered with thick purulent secretions of mucus. The lesion may be very painful, or the patient may have few symptoms. Tubercular fistulas are usually multiple.

The differential diagnosis for anoperineal TB is primarily Crohn's disease, which has remarkable clinical similarities with mycobacterial infections. Other possible granulomatous diseases of the anus to be considered are amoebiasis, sarcoidosis, syphilis, venereal lymphogranuloma with *Chlamydia trachomatis*, and cancer.

16.4 Pilonidal Sinus

Pilonidal sinus disease (PSD) is a disease of young people, usually men, which can result in an abscess. It probably results from hair penetration beneath the skin, for reasons that are not clear. A pilonidal sinus in the sacrococcygeal region is associated with recurrent infection, abscess formation, cellulitis, and fistulas. The infection is usually chronic and non-specific [8]. It typically occurs in the intergluteal region. Chronic PSD is treated with a wide excision and primary closure or secondary healing. The surgeon must know the dimensions, location, borders, and branches of the pilonidal sinus cavity in order to plan the operative strategy.

Palpation and methylene blue injection are typically used to estimate the borders of diseased tissue; however, most operative findings do not match the actual borders. Imaging methods, such as ultrasound, may therefore be useful to obtain a more accurate estimate of the size and margins of the lesion.

Perianal ultrasound reveals an intradermal hypoechoic lesion sometimes with internal echoic foci. When employed preoperatively while deciding upon the correct surgical intervention for PSD, perianal ultrasound can improve the identification of the sinus tract, its borders, and its branches compared to palpation and methylene blue injection.

As reported by Mentes et al. [9] in a prospective study evaluating the borders, opening, and location of the sinus tract, the use of ultrasonography prior to surgery correctly identified the borders of the sinus tissue, which were similar to the borders marked by the surgeon, in 56 of 73 patients (76.6%). Importantly, however, in the remaining 17 patients (23.3%), perianal ultrasonography detected branches or borders that distinctly exceeded the planned incision line, thus changing the surgical plan in these patients.

16.5 Perianal Actinomycosis

Actinomycotic anal infection of cryptoglandular origin is a specific and extremely rare cause of anal suppuration. Its recognition is important because surgical treatment and specific antibiotic therapy are mandatory to achieve complete eradication and to avoid multiple inappropriate surgical procedures. Actinomycosis, despite its rarity, should be considered in the spectrum of disorders involving the anorectal region (acute abscess, chronic abscess, fistula, rectal stenosis mimicking carcinomatosis) in immunocompetent populations but also in HIV-infected patients [10].

Actinomycosis should be suspected particularly in cases of indolent anal suppuration. Careful histological examination of the excised tissue and appropriate anaerobic cultures of pus should be carried out to ultimately achieve complete eradication of this seldom occurring but easily curable disease. The first-line antibiotic in anal actinomycosis is penicillin or a penicillin-related antibiotic.

References

1. Pfenninger JL, Zainea GG (2001) Common anorectal conditions: Part II. Lesions. Am Fam Physician 64:77-88
2. Christison-Lagay ER, Hall JF, Wales PW, et al (2007). Nonoperative management of perianal abscess in infants is associated with decreased risk for fistula formation. Pediatrics 120:e548-52
3. 3.Wiseman MC (2004) Hidradenitis suppurativa: a review Dermatol Ther 17:50-4
4. Roy MK, Appleton MAC, Delicata RJ, et al (1997) .Probable association between hidradenitis suppurativa and Crohn's disease: significance of epithelioid granuloma. Br J Surg 84:375-376
5. Wortsman X, Gregor BEJ (2007) Real-time compound imaging ultrasound of hidradenitis suppurativa. Dermatol Surg 33:1340-1342
6. Kelekis NL, Efstathopoulos E, Balanika A, et al (2010) Ultrasound aids in diagnosis and severity assessment of hidradenitis suppurativa. Br J Dermatol 162:1400-1402
7. Sultan S, Azria F, Bauer P, et al (2002) Anoperineal tuberculosis: diagnostic and management considerations in seven cases. Dis Colon Rectum 45:407-10
8. Gupta PJ (2012) Pilonidal sinus disease and tuberculosis. Eur Rev Med Pharmacol Sci 16:19-24
9. Mentes O, Oysul A, Harlak A et al (2009) Ultrasonography accurately evaluates the dimension and shape of the pilonidal sinus. Clinics (Sao Paulo) 64:189-92
10. Bauer P, Sultan S, Atienza P (2006) Perianal actinomycosis: diagnostic and management considerations: a review of six cases. Gastroenterol Clin Biol 30:29-32

Artifacts and Pitfalls

17

Giovanni Maconi, Cristina Bezzio and Giulio A. Santoro

17.1 Introduction

As discussed elsewhere in this volume, transanal ultrasound is a simple, rapid and minimally invasive procedure that can accurately detect and classify perianal fistulas and their complications. It is also useful to monitor patients after treatment, to guide their management. To date, the scientific literature is generally positive regarding the usefulness of transanal and transperineal ultrasound in assessing perianal disease. However, it is also well known that the magnitude of accuracy of these techniques may vary, depending on the complexity of perianal disease considered in the published series and the expertise of the investigators, since transanal and transperineal ultrasound are operator-dependent procedures; both are therefore vulnerable to pitfalls and have specific disadvantages, considered below.

The well recognised advantage of transanal ultrasound is its high spatial resolution, which allows precise definition of the sphincter muscle complex and delineation of the internal opening of a perianal fistula. This property, mainly relevant to high-frequency ultrasound, is particularly useful for structures and lesions closer to the rectal probe, where imaging and thus the investigation are more accurate and precise; however, it constitutes a limit for lesions that lie far from the probe, which are accordingly less accurately imaged and more frequently misinterpreted or missed.

The insufficient penetration of the ultrasound beam beyond the external sphincter, especially with high-frequency transducers, restricts the physician's

G. Maconi (✉)
Gastroenterology Unit, Department of Biomedical and Clinical Sciences
Luigi Sacco University Hospital
Milan, Italy
e-mail: giovanni.maconi@unimi.it

M.Tonolini and G. Maconi (eds.), *Imaging of Perianal Inflammatory Diseases*,
DOI: 10.1007/978-88-470-2847-0_17, © Springer-Verlag Italia 2013

ability to resolve ischioanal and supralevator infections, with the result that extensions and complications from the primary tract into these sites (e.g., in the perirectal space or near the scrotum or vagina) may be missed.

17.2 Overcoming the Limitations of Transanal Ultrasound

Deep internal extensions and complications are a challenge and sometimes an unavoidable limitation for ultrasound. Thus, alternative ultrasonographic approaches such as transvaginal ultrasound and transabdominal ultrasound may, under favorable conditions (e.g. thin patients), yield more useful information. Superficial extensions and complications not detectable by transanal ultrasound may be better imaged using transperineal ultrasound, which due to its simplicity and wide availability is a quite useful method to investigate suspected fistulous lesions in or near the gluteus, scrotum, or labia in order to assess their anal connection and confirm their fistulous nature (Fig. 17.1).

To overcome the poor visualization of fistulous tracts, clarify the course of patent tracts, and correctly classify perianal fistulas, hydrogen peroxide transanal ultrasound is frequently used [1-3]. However, this procedure does not avoid the risks of misinterpretation. In fact, after the injection of hydrogen peroxide into the external opening, gas within the tract may produce shadowing that mimics extensions. This phenomenon can occur with any tract that contains air, leading, for example, to intersphincteric fistulas being inadvertently classified as transsphincteric (Fig. 17.2). Similarly, when the exter-

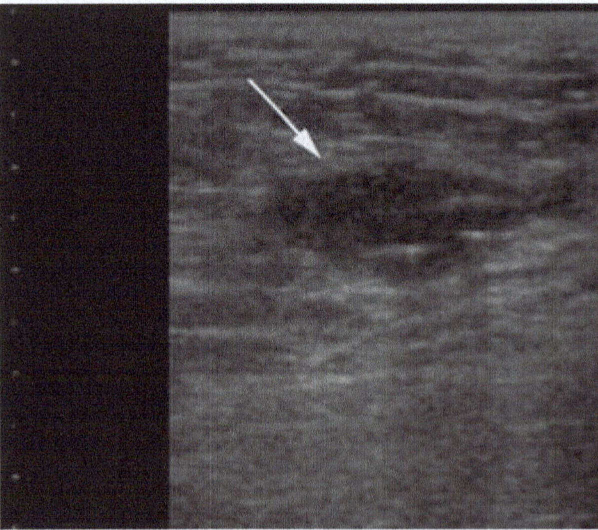

Fig. 17.1 A small superficial abscess (*arrow*) in the gluteal subcutaneous tissues that was not detectable by transanal ultrasound but imaged using transperineal ultrasound

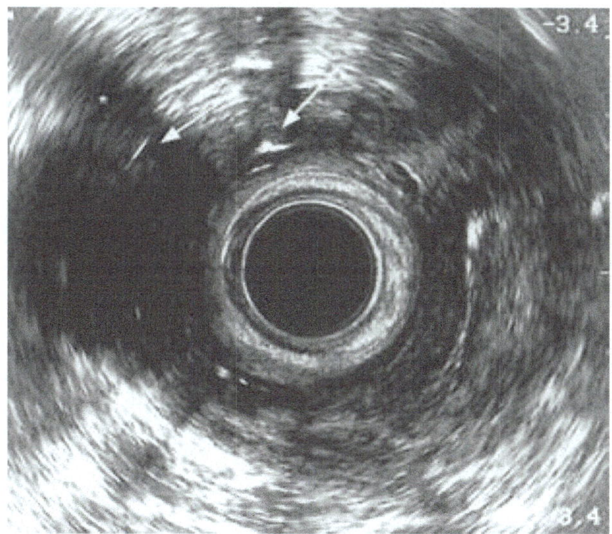

Fig. 17.2 Transverse transanal sonogram at the upper anal canal level, showing intersphincteric horseshoe extension (*arrows*). Gas in the fistula causes acoustic shadowing, which could be mistaken for a transsphincteric tract

nal opening is close to the anal opening and it is difficult to detect the presence of severe perianal disease, indurations, and skin tags, hydrogen peroxide may leak from the external opening across the skin and reflux into the anal canal and the rectum, thus hampering sonographic visualization in addition to mimicking at transperianal examination the presence of an intasphincteric or complex fistula. In fact, air in the anal canal, in particular in patients with anal ulcers, has an appearance similar to that of hydrogen peroxide and results in brightly echogenic shadowing that seems to arise from the lumen of the anal canal, suggesting a patent tract communicating with the anal lumen. Likewise, setons, surgical sutures, and hemorrhoidal bands in the anal wall should be identified before hydrogen peroxide injection, because these are echogenic and may simulate gas within a fistula or small intramural abscesses (Fig. 17.3).

An exact ultrasonographic definition and classification of complex perianal fistulas and perianal abscesses may be limited using bi-dimensional evaluation. Transanal ultrasound and transperineal ultrasound are disadvantaged by their inability to image the coronal and transversal planes, respectively. Therefore, using conventional transanal ultrasound it is difficult to distinguish supra- from infralevator extensions and abscesses (Fig 17.4). Likewise, assessment of the internal opening of a fistula is more difficult using transperineal ultrasound, in particular for complex fistulas (supra- or extrasphincteric fistulas), also due to the limited penetration of the ultrasonographic beam. To overcome this disadvantage, transanal ultrasound is usually performed with three-dimensional acquisitions [4].

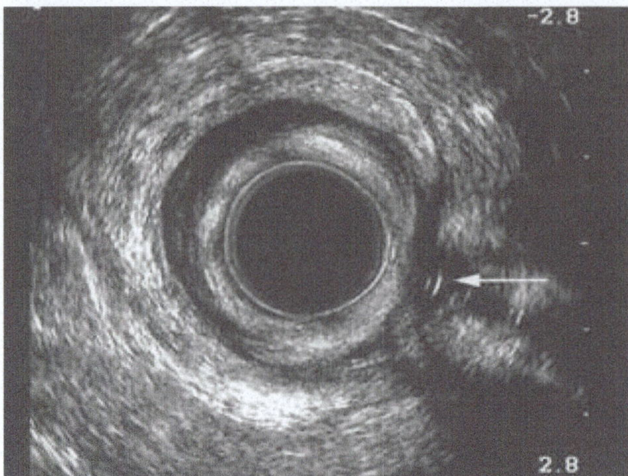

Fig. 17.3 Transanal sonogram at the level of the upper anal canal, showing a seton within the fistula (*arrow*)

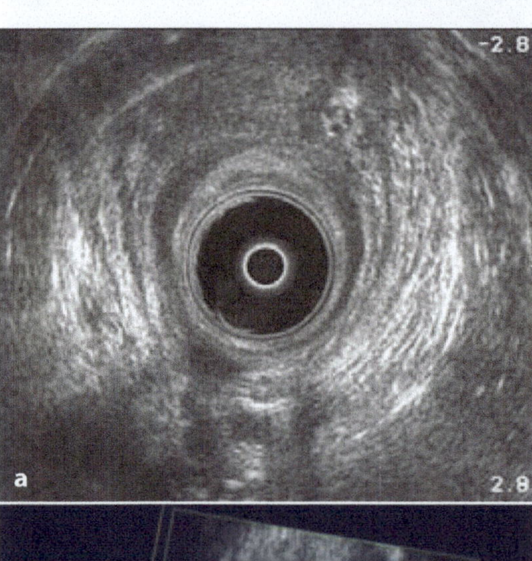

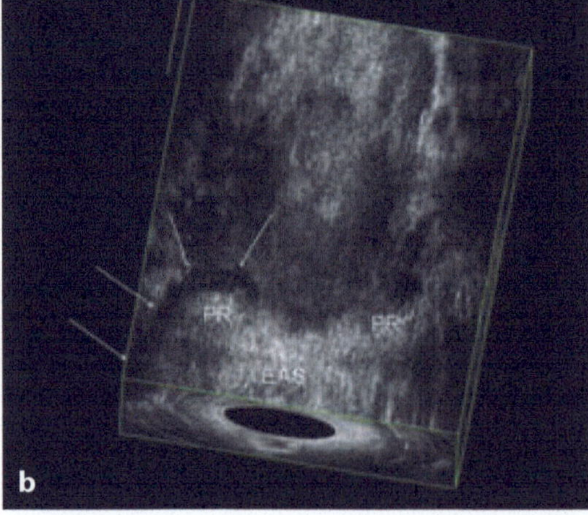

Fig. 17.4 a Transanal sonogram showing a fistula that based on the initial 2D image was classified as transsphincteric. **b** After a 3-D sonogram, the same fistula was newly classified as suprasphincteric with supralavator extension. Courtesy of Prof. Giulio A. Santoro, from [8]

Another limit of ultrasound is its difficulty in distinguishing active from inactive or fibrotic fistulous tracts, and sometimes collections from active fistulas.

Active fistulas and inactive fistulas both may have a hypoechoic appearance; in some patients with recurrent perianal disease, active tracts and fibrotic scars may coexist. In this context, visual ability to judge activity using gray-scale echogenicity is hampered and may be influenced by the brightness and shadowing of surrounding structures. Instead, a quantitative computerized analysis of digitalized images of fistulas has been suggested, but this is time-consuming and thus far impractical. However, the use of intravenous contrast-enhanced ultrasound during transanal or transperineal ultrasound, by depicting vascularization in the perianal fistulas and masses, could significantly improve the detection of perianal abscesses and accurately distinguish vascularized fistulas from non-vascularized collections. Nonetheless, to date, these methods have not been tested in clinical trials and their accuracy compared with MRI or surgical examination remains to be assessed.

Finally, as previously stated, transanal ultrasound and perianal ultrasound are operator-dependent procedures. Although a specific learning curve for the ultrasonographic detection of perianal inflammatory diseases has not been determined, previous studies have shown that transanal ultrasound is a simple procedure to learn and that, once a moderate degree of experience is gained (30 examinations), it could be routinely incorporated into the evaluation of rectal cancer, based on an accuracy > 75% [5, 6]. In transperineal ultrasound, experienced abdominal sonographers achieve competency at performing anal canal evaluation after approximately 12 patients [7].

References

1. Buchanan GN, Bartram CI, Williams AB, et al (2005) Value of hydrogen peroxide enhancement of three-dimensional endoanal ultrasound in fistula-in-ano. Dis Colon Rectum 48:141-7
2. Poen AC, Felt-Bersma RJ, Eijsbouts QA, et al (1998) Hydrogen peroxide-enhanced transanal ultrasound in the assessment of fistula-in-ano. Dis Colon Rectum 41:1147-52
3. Navarro-Luna A, Garcia-Domingo MI, Rius-Macias J, et al (2004) Ultrasound study of anal fistulas with hydrogen peroxide enhancement. Dis Colon Rectum 47:108-14
4. West RL, Dwarkasing S, Schouten WR, et al (2004) Hydrogen peroxide-enhanced three-dimensional endoanal ultrasonography and endoanal magnetic resonance imaging in evaluating perianal fistulas: agreement and patient preference. Eur J Gastroenterol Hepatol 16:1319-24
5. Carmody BJ, Otchy DP (2000) Learning curve of transrectal ultrasound. Dis Colon Rectum 43:193-7
6. Badger SA, Devlin PB, Neilly PJ, Gilliland R (2007) Preoperative staging of rectal carcinoma by endorectal ultrasound: is there a learning curve? Int J Colorectal Dis 22:1261-8
7. Stewart LK, McGee J, Wilson SR (2001) Transperineal and transvaginal sonography of perianal inflammatory disease. AJR Am J Roentgenol 177:627-32
8. Santoro GA, Di Falco G (2006) Benign Anorectal Diseases. Springer, Milan

Section V

Magnetic Resonance Imaging

MRI Study Protocol

18

Alessandro Campari and Massimo Tonolini

18.1 Technique and Equipment

Focused MRI of the anus and perianal region should be performed on high-magnetic-field scanners operating at 1–1.5 T. Acquisition using 1.5-T clinical equipment is recommended but (as our experience confirms) a 1.0-T scanner is adequate, although it does pose disadvantages in terms of the duration of the exam [1].

In the 1990s, the first reports of MRI examination of the perianal region described the adoption of the body coil integrated in the MR scanner, allowing for a large field-of-view (FOV). However, the spatial resolution was insufficient, thus limiting diagnostic accuracy [2]. At the beginning of the 21st century, the introduction of endorectal coils provided very high spatial resolution and thus a very detailed view of the limited perianal region as well as an accurate depiction of internal fistulous openings. Nonetheless, there were significant drawbacks to this technique, including complex patient preparation, technical difficulties in patients with anal pain or stenosis, and poor examination tolerance, often resulting in motion artifacts. Perhaps more importantly, the limited FOV resulted in an incomplete visualization of complex perianal Crohn's disease [2-4].

Following further technological evolution and the above considerations, most centers adopted phased-array MRI coils as the accepted standard in clinical practice. This approach offered a reasonable compromise between a large-enough FOV to assess disease extending towards the levator ani muscle and sufficient spatial resolution to allow the identification of the two sphincteric layers [1, 4, 5].

A. Campari (✉)
Diagnostic and Interventional Radiology Department
San Paolo Hospital – University of Milan
Milan, Italy
e-mail: alessandro.campari@unimi.it

M.Tonolini and G. Maconi (eds.), *Imaging of Perianal Inflammatory Diseases*,
DOI: 10.1007/978-88-470-2847-0_18, © Springer-Verlag Italia 2013

18.2 Patient Preparation and Positioning

Patients scheduled for perianal MRI are advised to fast for several hours before the examination, but no special bowel preparation is needed. Ideally, the urinary bladder should be moderately distended. Most centers do not routinely administer antispastic medications (particularly N-butylscopolamine), considering the limited occurrence of peristalsis-related artifacts in the pelvic region [6].

Patients are scanned in the supine position, with a phased-array coil precisely centered at the level of the pubic symphysis. Special attention should be paid by the radiology technician during coil application, since a more cranial positioning may result in an insufficient signal from structures of interest, such as the gluteal region [7].

18.3 Acquisition Protocol

Ideally, the MRI study should be performed according to a standardized protocol in order to maximize reproducibility, thus allowing for a precise comparison during follow-up studies [8]. Typical imaging protocols on 1.0 T and 1.5 T MRI scanners are summarized in Tables 18.1 and 18.2. They have been adopted by our centers.

Initial acquisition of a sagittally oriented T2-weighted turbo- or fast-spin echo (TSE/FSE) sequence provides a panoramic view of both the urogenital structures and the anorectal tract. The anal canal should be identified on the midline sagittal T2-weighted image. This will allow precise planning of the subsequent axial and coronal sequences oriented along oblique planes perpendicularly and parallel to the longitudinal axis, respectively (Fig. 18.1) [1, 6].

High-resolution T2-weighted images acquired with a limited FOV allow differentiation of the two sphincter components, as the internal sphincter has a slightly higher signal intensity than the external one, in which the signal is comparable to that of the levator ani and other muscles. The normal, fat-containing intersphincteric space will usually have a very thin imaging appearance. Furthermore, T2-weighted imaging provides the intrinsic soft-tissue contrast needed to identify fistulas, abscesses, and scar tissue. Coronal images are required to identify the levator ani and thus to differentiate between the supralevator, ischiorectal, and ischioanal spaces [5].

A large-FOV axial fat-suppressed sequence may be useful to provide a panoramic view of the pelvis, including its bony structures, the bladder, female genital organs, and the presacral space, with easy appreciation of edematous tissues and fluid structures. Fat suppression or STIR technique may result in significant interpretation uncertainty due to the reduced conspicuity of normal anatomical landmarks and to the relatively high signal of certain normal structures such as the prostate and the periprostatic and vaginal vessels; indeed, the majority of experienced readers rely mostly on high-resolution T2 images [5, 6].

Table 18.1 MRI acquisition protocols on a 1-T clinical MRI scanner

Sequence	1	2	3	4	5 Optional	Contrast medium administration	6	7	8
	T2 TSE	T2 TSE	T2 TSE	STIR	T1 TSE		T1 SPIR	T1 TSE	T1 TSE
Plane	Sagittal	Axial	Coronal	Axial	Axial		Axial	Coronal	Sagittal
FOV (mm)	320	220	250	300	220		220	250	250
TR/TE (ms)	3600/90	3500/90	4500/90	1972/15	522/13		999/13	668/14	668/14
TI (ms)				155					
Thickness (mm)	6	3	6	5	4		4	6	6
Gap (mm)	0.6	1	0.6	1	0.4		0.4	0.6	0.6
NEX	3	3	3	3	4		4	2-3	2-3
Slices	20	30	25	30	30		30	25	20
Time	1' 20"	4' 10"	1' 40"	2' 52"	3' 45"		7'	2' 24"	2' 24"

Table 18.2 MRI acquisition protocols on a 1.5-T clinical MRI scanner

Sequence	1	2	3	4 Optional	5 Optional			6	7 Optional
	T2 TSE	T2 TSE Fat suppression	T2 TSE	T2 TSE Fat suppression	DWI	Contrast medium administration	50-s delay	T1 TSE Fat suppression	T1 TSE Fat suppression
Plane	Axial	Axial	Coronal	Coronal	Axial			Axial	Coronal
FOV (mm)	200	200	200	200	230			200	200
TR/TE (ms)	5670/108	6290/108	5670/108	6290/108	1707/78				
B values					50 - 500 - 1000				
Thickness (mm)	3	3	3	3	5			4	4
Gap (mm)	1	1	1	1	1			2	2
Slices	30	30	20	20	30			30	20
Time	2’	2-3’	2-3’	2-3’	3-4’			3-4’	3-4’

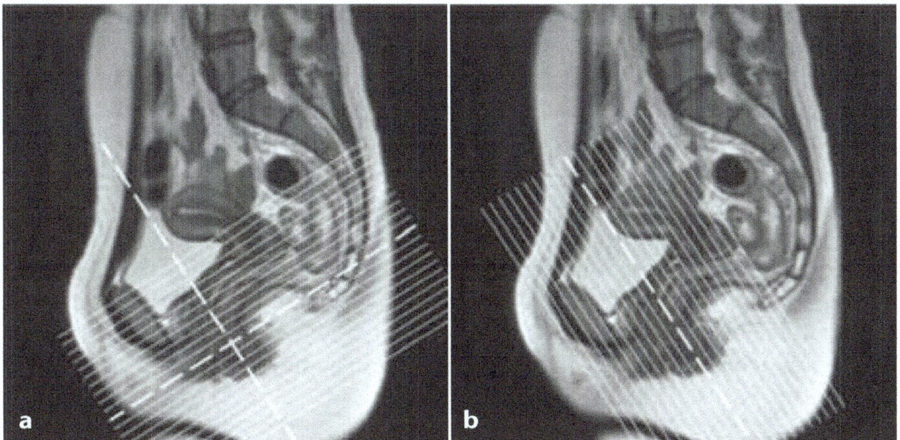

Fig. 18.1 Midline sagittal T2-weighted imaging allows identification of the longitudinal axis of the anal canal (usually inclined 30–40° from the vertical) and the orientation of axial (**a**) and coronal (**b**) images, respectively, perpendicular and parallel

A combined assessment of axial and coronal images facilitates the classification of perianal inflammatory disease according to the relationships with the two sphincteric layers and the intersphincteric and ischioanal spaces. Correlation with sagittal images is needed when checking for the anovaginal septum or for presacral space involvement.

The acquisition of pre-contrast T1-weighted sequences is considered optional by most authors since in most cases it does not offer additional diagnostic information, even though T1 imaging may be useful in the postoperative setting to identify recent hemorrhage or fat-containing grafts [6].

The vast majority of MRI centers routinely acquire post-contrast T1-weighted sequences after the injection of standard-dose paramagnetic gadolinium-based contrast, such as 0.2 mmol/kg Gd-DTPA (MagneVist, Schering) or gadoterate (Dotarem, alternatively 0.1 mmol/kg Gd-BOPTA – MultiHance, Bracco – or gadobutrol – GadoVist, Schering). After intravenous contrast, suppression of background fat with SPIR (spectral presaturation with inversion recovery) or similar techniques greatly helps visual recognition of active disease, since inflamed granulation tissue in the walls of abscess and fistulas enhances whereas chronic fistulas usually do not, and fluid in tracts and the contents of purulent abscesses remain T1-hypointense [5].

Globally, an acquisition time of 20–25 min should be expected for a comprehensive MRI examination of the perianal region [6].

18.4 Additional Investigations and Future Developments

Recently, diffusion-weighted imaging (DWI) with single-shot echo-planar acquisition has been investigated. Its implementation was found to increase diagnostic confidence compared to the interpretation of T2-weighted images alone. The same authors proposed DWI as a useful adjunct sequence particularly in patients with contraindications or risk factors for intravenous contrast [9].

Detection of thin anovaginal fistulas can be improved by the injection of saline [10] or diluted gadolinium (1:10 in saline solution) into the fistulous opening (direct MR-fistulography technique) [4] or by the application of a small volume of diluted gadolinium-containing rectal enema (indirect MR-fistulography technique), but these methods are cumbersome and should be reserved for very selected cases [11].

References

1. Szurowska E, Wypych J, Izycka-Swieszewska E (2007) Perianal fistulas in Crohn's disease: MRI diagnosis and surgical planning : MRI in fistulizing perianal Crohn's disease. Abdom Imaging 32:705-718
2. Halligan S, Stoker J (2006) Imaging of fistula in ano. Radiology 239:18-33
3. Beets-Tan RG, Beets GL, van der Hoop AG, et al. (2001) Preoperative MR imaging of anal fistulas: Does it really help the surgeon? Radiology 218:75-84
4. Maccioni F, Colaiacomo MC, Stasolla A, et al (2002) Value of MRI performed with phased-array coil in the diagnosis and pre-operative classification of perianal and anal fistulas. Radiol Med 104:58-67
5. Horsthuis K, Stoker J (2004) MRI of perianal Crohn's disease. AJR Am J Roentgenol 183:1309-1315
6. Torkzad MR, Karlbom U (2011) MRI for assessment of anal fistula. Insights Imaging 1:62-71
7. Laniado M, Makowiec F, Dammann F, et al. (1997) Perianal complications of Crohn disease: MR imaging findings. Eur Radiol 7:1035-1042
8. Bell SJ, Halligan S, Windsor AC, et al (2003) Response of fistulating Crohn's disease to infliximab treatment assessed by magnetic resonance imaging. Aliment Pharmacol Ther 17:387-393
9. Hori M, Oto A, Orrin S, et al (2009) Diffusion-weighted MRI: a new tool for the diagnosis of fistula in ano. J Magn Reson Imaging 30:1021-1026
10. Myhr GE, Myrvold HE, Nilsen G, et al (1994) Perianal fistulas: use of MR imaging for diagnosis. Radiology 191:545-549
11. Ergen FB, Arslan EB, Kerimoglu U, et al (2007) Magnetic resonance fistulography for the demonstration of anovaginal fistula: an alternative imaging technique? J Comput Assist Tomogr 31:243-246

Dynamic MRI and the Assessment of Activity

19

Chiara Villa

19.1 Dynamic MRI

Paramagnetic contrast administration is routinely used in the evaluation of perianal disease in order to detect the presence of active inflammation within fistula tracts as well as abscesses.

Spencer et al. were the first to propose the use of dynamic contrast-enhanced MRI sequences to assess the presence of active inflammation in perianal fistulas. They found that contrast-active tracts showed vivid enhancement compared to the lower signal intensity of healed tracts. Indeed, MRI including contrast-enhanced sequences was able to provide pathologic information in addition to an accurate morphological study [1]. Since that initial report, all recent reviews of the role of MRI in the study of perianal disease have recommended the use of gadolinium [2-7]. Horsthuis et al. studied the role of dynamic contrast-enhanced MRI in determining the disease activity of fistulas. They concluded that a rapid uptake of gadolinium correlated with more severe disease than indicated by the patient's perianal disease activity index (PDAI) [8]. A more recent study demonstrated a highly significant association between the absence of enhancement and clinical remission. Indeed, the disappearance of contrast enhancement was the only MRI feature associated with remission [9].

In our practice, after paramagnetic contrast agent injection, transverse and coronal SPIR (spectral presaturation with inversion recovery) T1-weighted sequences are acquired during the following seven minutes. Dynamic contrast-enhanced gradient-echo sequences are not performed, based on the reduced

C. Villa (✉)
Radiology Department, Luigi Sacco University Hospital
Milan, Italy
e-mail: chiara.villa@hotmail.it

M.Tonolini and G. Maconi (eds.), *Imaging of Perianal Inflammatory Diseases*,
DOI: 10.1007/978-88-470-2847-0_19, © Springer-Verlag Italia 2013

spatial resolution achieved by the MR scanner compared to the good signal-to-noise ratio obtained using spin-echo sequences. Moreover, the analysis of dynamic contrast-enhanced images requires further MRI data elaboration, which is not feasible on every MRI workstation.

Previous color and power-Doppler ultrasound analysis in patients with Crohn's disease (CD) showed that the vessel density in the affected bowel loops reflects disease activity and that recognition of a pathologically increased vascularization within internal or perianal fistulas or abscesses identifies acute inflammatory conditions [10-12]. It is therefore useful to quantify the degree of vascularization of perianal fistulas in patients with CD by administering gadoliniumin in order to monitor disease activity.

Contrast enhancement of a fistula can be quantitatively assessed using the protocol recently proposed by Villa et al. [13]. The most enhancing sections of the middle tract of the fistula on preliminary visual analysis are chosen and

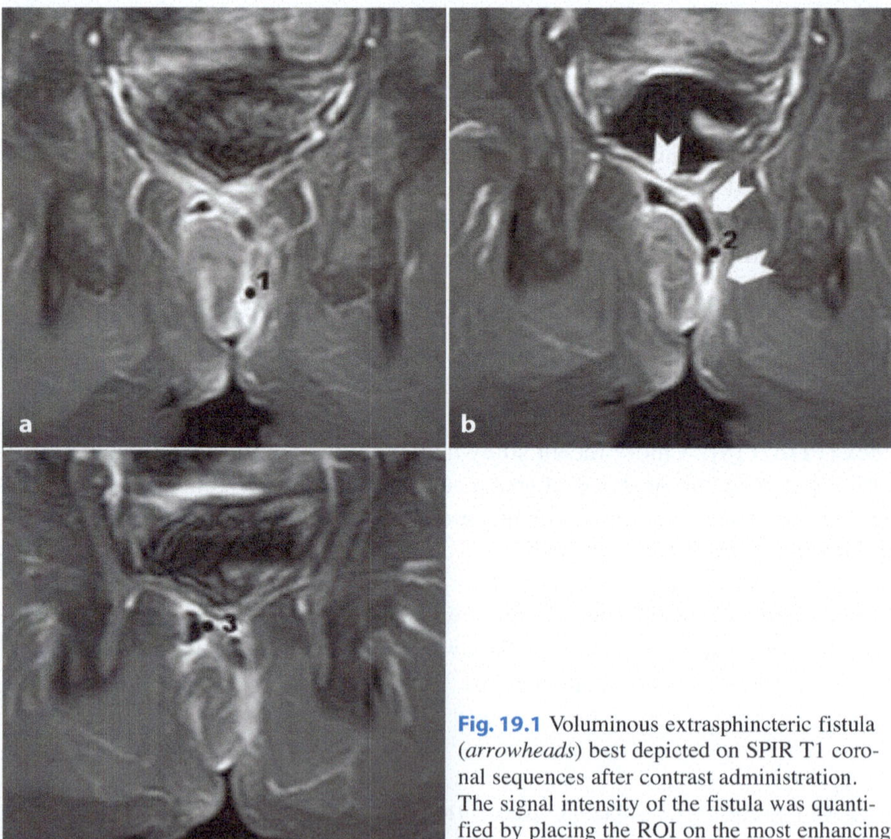

Fig. 19.1 Voluminous extrasphincteric fistula (*arrowheads*) best depicted on SPIR T1 coronal sequences after contrast administration. The signal intensity of the fistula was quantified by placing the ROI on the most enhancing middle tract of the fistula, within the fistula's walls, as shown by *1*, *2* and *3*

three 2-mm^2 elliptical, manually drawn ROIs (regions of interest) are placed within the walls of the fistula (Fig. 19.1). For each ROI, the mean value is recorded; the average of these measurements, i.e., the quantified signal intensity of the fistula (S_f) after contrast administration, is then calculated. On the same sequences, three elliptical manually drawn ROI of 5 mm^2 are placed on different regions of the locoregional healthy fat, either of the ischioanal fossa or of the gluteus. The average of their mean values, i.e., the quantified signal intensity of the healthy fat (S_{hf}) after contrast administration, is similarly calculated (Fig. 19.2). The percentage increase (PI) in the signal intensity of the fistula compared to that of healthy fat is determined as: $PI = (S_f - S_{hf}) \times 100 / S_{hf}$. This value expresses the degree of contrast enhancement of the fistula relative to that of normal perianal tissue.

A significant association between the increase in the signal intensity of the fistula after contrast administration and the severity of perianal disease,

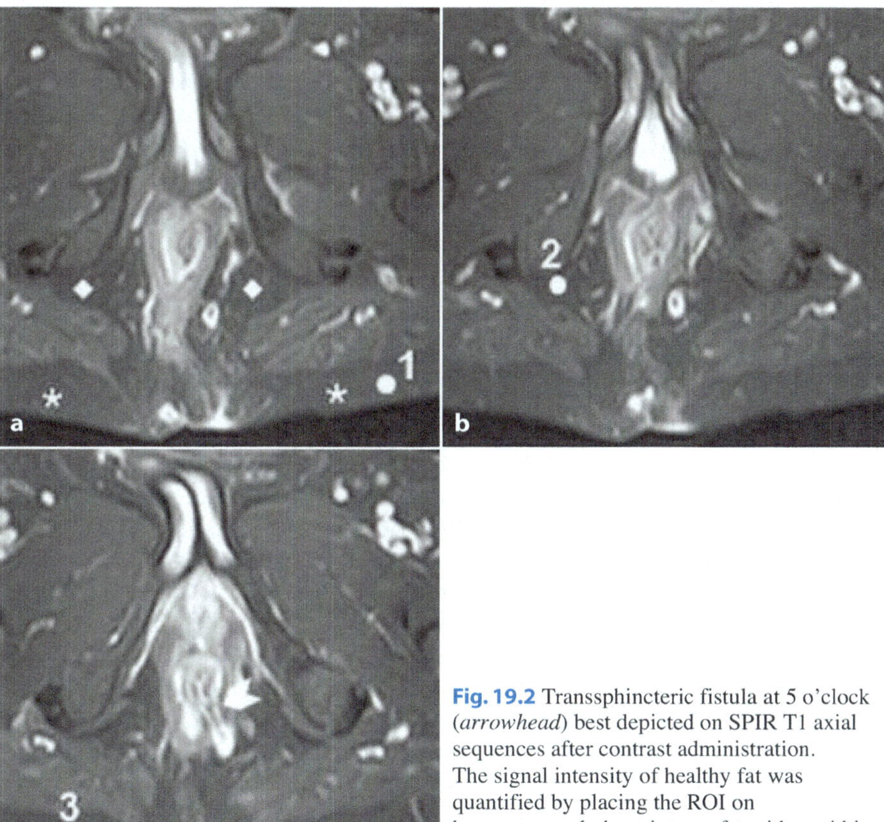

Fig. 19.2 Transsphincteric fistula at 5 o'clock (*arrowhead*) best depicted on SPIR T1 axial sequences after contrast administration. The signal intensity of healthy fat was quantified by placing the ROI on homogeneously hypointense fat, either within the gluteus (*) or the ischioanal fossa (◇), as shown by *1*, *2* and *3*

assessed by the PDAI and fistula drainage assessment (FDA), was reported. The PI thus appears to be of satisfactory diagnostic ability, offering a practical and immediate tool to quantify the degree of contrast enhancement of the fistula [10].

19.2 Assessment of Activity

Correct management in the follow-up of patients with fistula-related complications, which commonly include relapse, consists of contrast-enhanced MRI to assess the activity of perianal fistulas. As already demonstrated in previous studies [9, 14-18], MRI yields useful information regarding changes in the internal aspects of the fistula tract during long-term medical therapy and can demonstrate persistent disease activity despite healing of the external orifices and cessation of the fistula's drainage. It is therefore mandatory to quantify disease activity within the walls of the fistula in order to monitor the healing process and prevent recurrences.

At our institute, for each fistula tract detected, a PI score, which offers a quantitative assessment of the degree of contrast enhancement of the fistula relative to that of normal perianal tissue, is calculated. This score provides a reliable indicator of the disease activity of the fistula [13]. As noted above, the diagnostic ability of the PI in discriminating between the presence of active inflammation and fibrosis within the fistula tract has been investigated with respect to the PDAI and FDA. A significant association between the PI and the severity of perianal disease as assessed by these clinical indices was determined.

Considering a PDAI score > 4 as the reference cut-off value in depicting clinically active perianal disease [19], a fair ability of PI as a diagnostic tool was demonstrated (ROC curve analysis, AUC = 0.876). The diagnostic ability of PI in estimating disease activity according to the FDA score of active or inactive disease is also satisfactory (ROC curve analysis, AUC = 0.784). Moreover, a PI threshold of 200 has been proposed to discriminate between active and inactive fistulas, showing a fair sensitivity and specificity (for PDAI and FDA, respectively, 93.8% and 71.4% and 97.7% and 58.3%), based on preliminary data.Examples of cases in which perianal fistulas were evaluated with the PI score are described in the following figures.

Figure 19.3 shows a voluminous intersphincteric horseshoe fistula (arrowhead) detected on axial T2-weighted sequences (Fig. 19.3a), seen as a diffuse hyperintense alteration within the posterior intersphincteric space on both sides and more evident on SPIR T2 sequences (Fig. 19.3b). On axial SPIR T1 sequences acquired after contrast administration (Fig. 19.3d), the fistula tract is well-delineated and shows vivid hyperintense signal compared to the same sequences before contrast (Fig. 19.3c), suggesting strong contrast enhancement. The mean ROI values measured within the walls of the fistula and within healthy local gluteal fat were, respectively, 1924 and 370. The PI score was

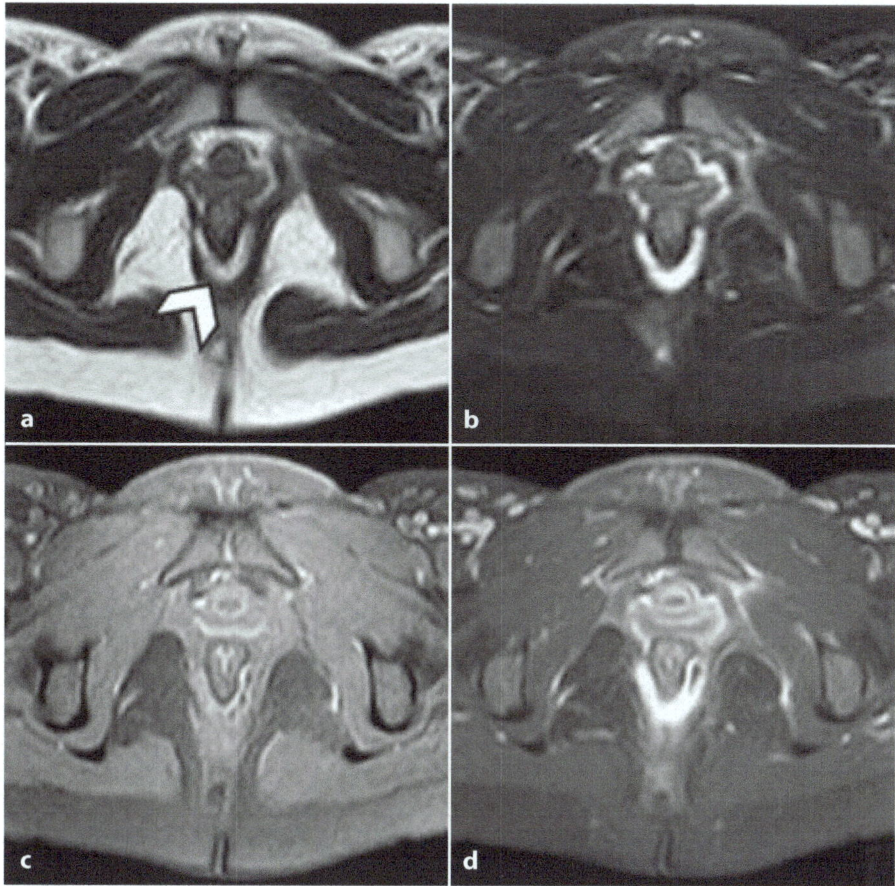

Fig. 19.3 Horseshoe intersphincteric fistula. **a** T2 axial sequence; **b** T2 SPIR axial sequence; **c** T1 SPIR axial sequence; **d** T1 SPIR axial sequence after contrast administration

420, indicating disease activity with respect to the PI threshold considered. These data were in agreement with the patient's PDAI score of 8 and an active FDA score.

The patient was started on anti-tumor-necrosis-factor (TNF)-α therapy maintenance and 1 year later underwent a further MRI examination (Fig. 19.4). At the time of the second examination, the patient did not have perianal discharge but reported mild pain and restriction in the usual daily activities. No external orifice was detected at clinical examination. The PDAI score was 5.

As seen on the follow-up images, the fistula tract is larger than on the previous examination, mostly on the left side (arrowheads). In addition, the suppurative component has increased, present as a hyperintense fluid alteration on

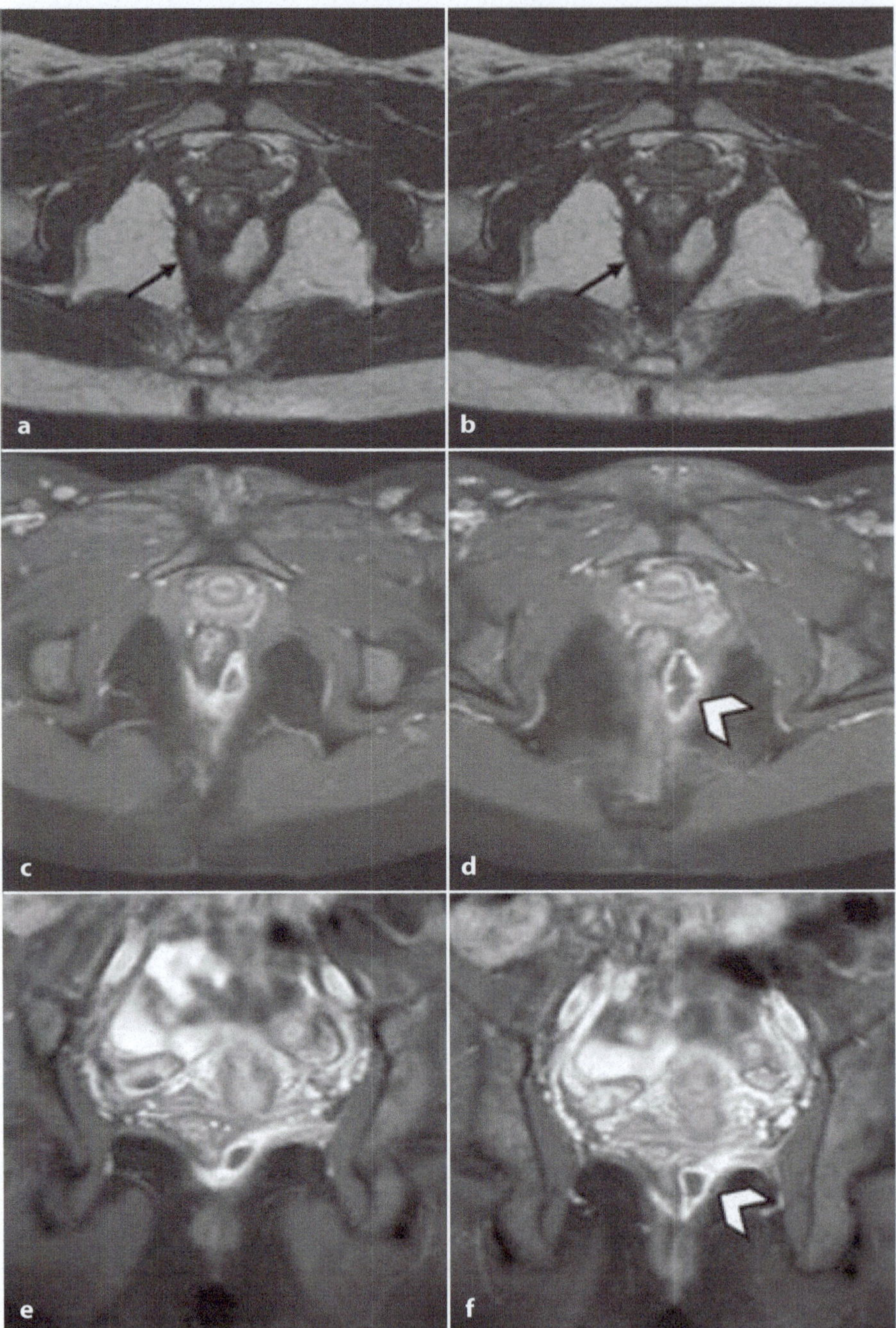

Fig. 19.4 Horseshoe intersphincteric fistula, control after one year. **a**, **b** T2 axial sequence; **c**, **d** T1 SPIR axial sequences after intravenous contrast administration; **e**, **f** T1 SPIR coronal sequences after intravenous contrast administration

the axial T2-weighted sequences (Fig. 19.4a). Axial and coronal SPIR T1 sequences acquired after contrast administration show a peripheral rim of contrast enhancement (Fig. 19.4b, c). T2 sequences show a reduction in the right side of the horseshoe fistula and in the hyperintense fluid component compared to the previous examination (Fig. 19.4a, black arrow). Contrast enhancement within the walls of the fistula on this side is also reduced (Fig. 19.4b, c). The mean ROI values measured within the walls of the fistula on the left and right sides and within healthy local gluteal fat were, respectively, 1110, 887, and 168. The PI score of the left side was 560, indicating an increase in disease activity and a recurrence, consistent with the morphological MRI finding of an enlarged suppurative component. The PI score on the right side was 427, which was not significantly different from that determined at the previous examina-

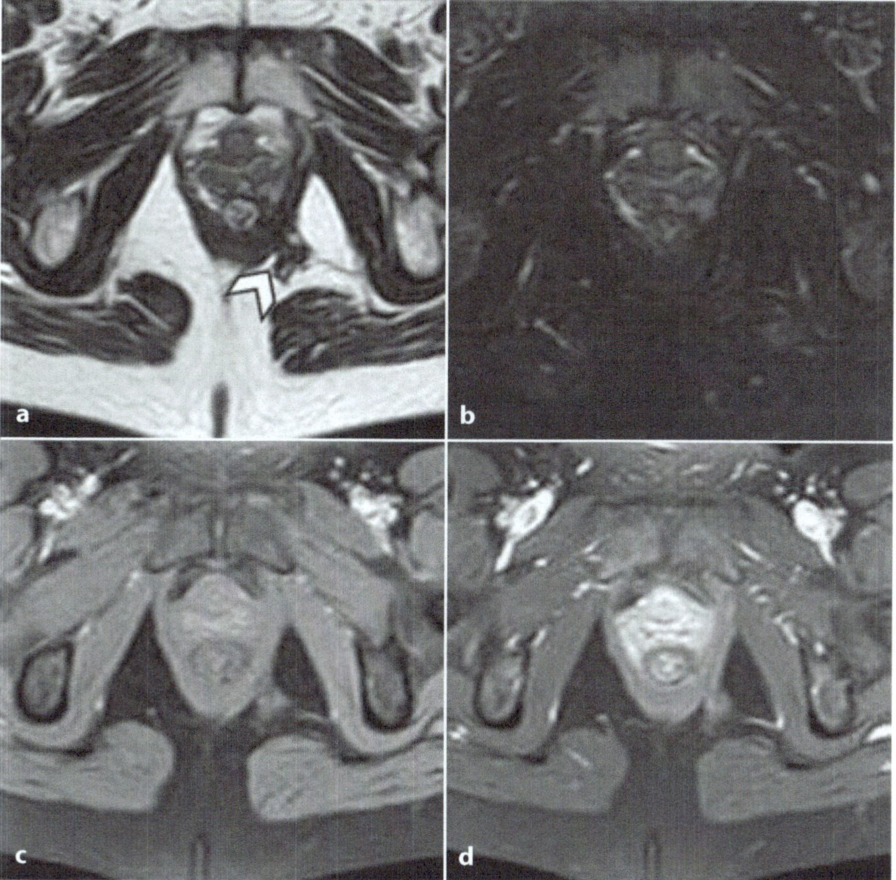

Fig. 19.5 Transsphincteric fistula at 4 o'clock. **a** T2 axial sequence; **b** T2 SPIR axial sequence; **c** T1 SPIR axial sequence; **d** T1 SPIR axial sequence after contrast administration

tion, indicating persistent disease activity even on this side, despite a decrease in both the fluid component and the thickness of the fistula. These data demonstrate that visual examination alone is not reliable in the evaluation of residual disease activity as seen on MRI contrast-enhanced sequences. Moreover, this case again highlights that, notwithstanding a decrease in the PDAI, there may be clinically silent recurrences. These should be always ruled out with scheduled MRI controls during the follow-up of medical treatment.

Figure 19.5 shows a transsphincteric fistula at 4 o'clock (arrowhead), detected on axial T2-weighted sequences (Fig. 19.5a) and seen as a short hypointense alteration involving both the internal and external anal sphincters, not evident on SPIR T2 sequences (Fig. 19.5b). On the axial SPIR T1 sequences acquired after contrast administration (Fig. 19.5d), the fistula tract does not show significant contrast enhancement compared to the T1 SPIR sequences acquired before contrast administration (Fig. 19.5c). The mean ROI values measured within the walls of the fistula and within healthy local fat of the contralateral ischioanal fossa were, respectively, 746 and 255. The PI score was 192, indicating inactive disease according to the PI threshold considered. The patient's PDAI was 3 and the FDA indicated inactive disease.

References

1. Spencer JA, Ward J, Beckingham IJ et al (1996) Dynamic contrast-enhanced MR imaging of perianal fistulas. AJR Am J Roentgenol 167:735-741
2. Morris J, Spencer JA, Ambrose NS (2000) MR imaging classification of perianal fistulas and its implications for patients management. Radiographics 20:623-637
3. Cuenod CA, de Parades V, Siauve N et al (2003) IRM des suppurations ano-périnéales. J Radiol 84:516-528
4. Dwarkasing S, Hussain SM, Krestin GP (2005) Magnetic resonance imaging of perianal fistulas. Semin Ultrasound CT MR 26:247-258
5. Halligan S, Stoker J (2006) Imaging of fistula in ano. Radiology 239:18-33
6. Sun MR, Smith MP, Kane RA (2008) Current techniques in imaging of fistula in ano: three-dimensional endoanal ultrasound and magnetic resonance imaging. Semin Ultrasound CT MR 29:454-471
7. Ziech M, Felt-Bersma R, Stoker J (2009) Imaging of perianal fistulas. Clin Gastroenterol Hepatol 7:1037-1045
8. Horsthuis K, Lavini C, Bipat S et al (2009) Perianal Crohn disease:evaluation of dynamic contrast-enhanced MR imaging as an indicator of disease activity. Radiology 251:380-387
9. Savoye-Collet C, Savoye G, Koning E et al (2010) Fistulizing perianal Crohn's disease: contrast-enhanced magnetic resonance imaging assessment at one year on maintenance anti-TNF-alpha therapy. Inflamm Bowel Dis 17(8):1751-1758.
10. Spalinger J, Patriquin H, Miron MC et al (2000) Doppler US in patients with Crohn disease: vessel density in the diseased bowel reflects disease activity. Radiology 217:787-791
11. Mallouhi A, Bonatti H, Peer S et al (2004) Detection and characterization of perianal inflammatory disease. J Ultrasound Med 23:19-27
12. Maconi G, Sampietro GM, Russo A et al (2002) The vascularity of internal fistulae in Crohn's disease: an in vivo power Doppler ultrasonography assessment. Gut 50(4):496-500
13. Villa C, Pompili G, Franceschelli G et al (2011) Role of magnetic resonance imaging in evaluation of the activity of perianal Crohn's disease. Eur J Radiol Feb 10

14. Bell SJ, Halligan S, Windsor AC et al (2003) Response of fistulating Crohn's disease to infliximab treatment assessed by magnetic resonance imaging. Aliment Pharmacol Ther 17:387-93
15. Van Assche G, Vanbeckevoort D, Bielen D et al (2003) Magnetic resonance imaging of the effects of infliximab on perianal fistulizing Crohn's disease. Am J Gastroenterol 98:332-339
16. Ng SC, Plamondon S, Gupta A et al (2009) Prospective evaluation of anti-tumor necrosis factor therapy guided by magnetic resonance imaging for Crohn's perineal fistulas. Am J Gastroenterol 104:2973-2986
17. Schwarts DA (2009) Imaging and the treatment of Crohn's perianal fistulas: to see is to believe. Am J Gastroenterol 104: 2987-2989
18. Karmiris K, Bielen D, Vanbeckevoort D et al (2011) Long-term monitoring of infliximab therapy for perianal fistulizing Crohn's disease by using magnetic resonance imaging. Clin Gastroenterol Hepatol. 9:130-136.
19. Losco A, Viganò C, Conte D et al (2009) Assessing the activity of perianal Crohn's disease: comparison of clinical indices and computer-assisted anal ultrasound. Inflamm Bowel Dis 15:742-749

Perianal Crohn's Disease MRI Classification and Staging

20

Francesca Maccioni, Giulia Bella and Valeria Buonocore

Perianal fistulas are a relatively frequent gastrointestinal pathology and an important cause of morbidity. They are particularly common in patients with Crohn's disease, who develop this complication in approximately 50% of cases [1, 2]. Fistulas frequently arise from the obstruction and infection of the anal crypts, in which the glands of Hermann and Desfosses flow, by feces, foreign bodies, or small local traumas. The fistulas may then spread towards the skin, within the rectal wall, or through the external sphincter towards the ischiorectal fossa.

20.1 Surgical Classifications of Anal/Perianal Fistulas

By definition, a fistula is an abnormal tract that connects two epithelial surfaces. The anatomic course of an anal fistula will be dictated by the location of the infected anal gland and the anatomic planes and boundaries that surround it. The radial positions of the fistula around the anus are referenced to a clock face, in which, according to the radiological classification, the 12 o'clock and 6 o'clock positions are, respectively, anteriorly and posteriorly directed [3].

Usually, the internal opening in the anal canal is located at the level of the dentate line, which is at the original site of the duct draining the infected gland. In most cases, this is located at the 6 o'clock position because the anal glands are more abundant posteriorly [4]. The fistula can reach the perianal skin by a variety of routes, some more tortuous than others, usually by variably penetrating and involving the muscles of the anal sphincter and surrounding tissues. Fistulas should be classified according to the route taken by the "primary tract" linking the internal and external openings.

F. Maccioni (✉)
Radiologic, Oncologic and Anatomopathologic Sciences, Policlinico Umberto I
Rome, Italy
e-mail: francesca.maccioni@uniroma1.it

M.Tonolini and G. Maconi (eds.), *Imaging of Perianal Inflammatory Diseases*,
DOI: 10.1007/978-88-470-2847-0_20, © Springer-Verlag Italia 2013

In 1934, Milligan and Morgan introduced the first classification of fistulas-in-ano based on the relationships between the tracts and the anorectal ring (anatomically, the puborectalis muscle). According to this early classification, anal fistulas were situated below the level of the ring whereas the anorectal type extended, at least partly, above the ring [5]. While this classification was subsequently modified and refined by other authors, the most comprehensive and practical classification, still in use today, is that of Parks et al., which is based on surgical findings [6]. Considering the external sphincter as the keystone, fistulas are classified into four main types and subtypes (Table 20.1, Fig. 20.1).

Type 1 fistulas (intersphincteric) (Figs. 20.1, 20.2) ramify only in the intersphincteric plane. This is the most common type and is sometimes known as the "low anal" fistula. It may be further subdivided into:

Table 20.1 Parks' classification (from [3])

Subcutaneous	No relation with the anal sphincter complex
Intersphincteric	Within the intersphincteric region, between the internal and external sphincters
Transsphincteric	Extends through both the internal and the external sphincter
Suprasphincteric	From the skin surface to the ischiorectal fossa, without communicating with the anal sphincter
Translevator	Above the levator ani muscle, within the pelvic region

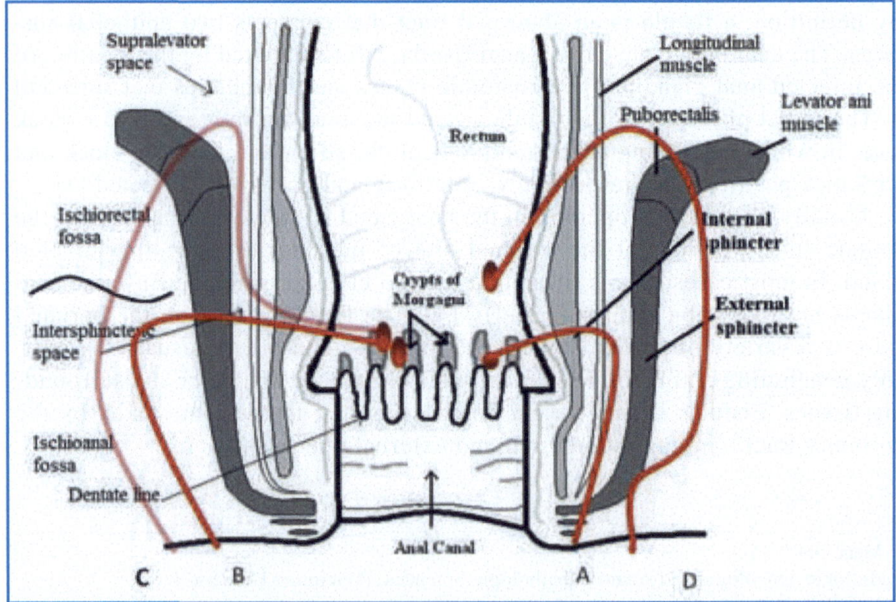

Fig. 20.1 The Parks classification of anal/perianal fistulas. *A* Intersphincteric fistula, *B* transsphincteric fistula, *C* suprasphincteric fistula, *D* extrasphincteric (translevator) fistula

- Simple intersphincteric fistula (Fig. 20.3). In this variety, the most common one, a tract passes from the primary abscess in the intersphincteric plane straight downwards to the anal verge.
- Intersphincteric fistula with a high blind tract. A is a high extension of the fistula between the internal sphincter and the longitudinal muscle of the upper anal canal passes upwards into the rectal wall itself.
- Intersphincteric fistula with a high tract opening into the lower rectum.
- High intersphincteric fistula without a perineal opening. The fistula commences in the intersphincteric zone of the mid-anal canal and passes upwards to end blindly in the rectal wall or to re-enter the rectum.
- High intersphincteric fistula with a pelvic extension. The tract passes upwards out into the pararectal space, instead of restricting its course to the rectal wall. There may or may not be a perineal opening.
- Intersphincteric fistula from pelvic disease. An infection from the pelvis can track downwards and reach the anal margin. In either case it pursues an intersphincteric course or it the may be extrasphincteric. This type is not a pure anal fistula at all, as its origin is completely outside defined area.

In **type 2 fistulas (transsphincteric)** (Figs. 20.4, 20.5) the tract passes from the intersphincteric plane through the external sphincter complex at varying levels into the ischiorectal fossa. Two subtypes are recognized:

- In uncomplicated cases, the tract passes from the intersphincteric plane of the mid-anal canal, through the external sphincter into the ischiorectal fossa and thence directly to the skin.
- In a transsphincteric fistula with a high blind tract, the tract crosses the external sphincter as previously described but then divides into two, giving rise to lower and upper halves. The lower tract passes to the perineal skin but the upper tract may reach the apex of the ischiorectal fossa or even higher, passing through the levator ani muscles into the true pelvic cavity.

In **type 3 fistulas (suprasphincteric)** (Fig. 20.6) the tract passes in the intersphincteric plane over the top of the puborectalis, then downwards again into the ischiorectal fossa and finally to the skin.

In **type 4 fistulas (extrasphincteric)** a tract passes from the perineal skin through the ischiorectal fat and levator muscles into the rectum (Fig. 20.7). This type is outside the external sphincter complex altogether. The following subtypes are recognized:

- In those secondary to a transsphincteric fistula, the tract from the latter passes upwards through the levator muscles to re-enter the rectum.
- In extrasphincteric fistulas due to trauma, there is direct communication between the rectum and the perineum.
- Extrasphincteric fistulas may also be due to a specific anorectal disease (inflammatory bowel disease or carcinoma).
- Alternatively, anextrasphincteric fistula may be due to pelvic inflammation, in which case an infection spreads downwards through the pelvic tissue, breaking through the levator ani muscles and emerging in the perineum.

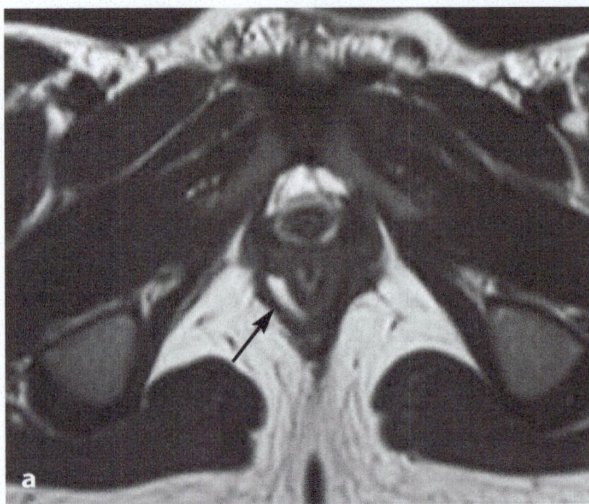

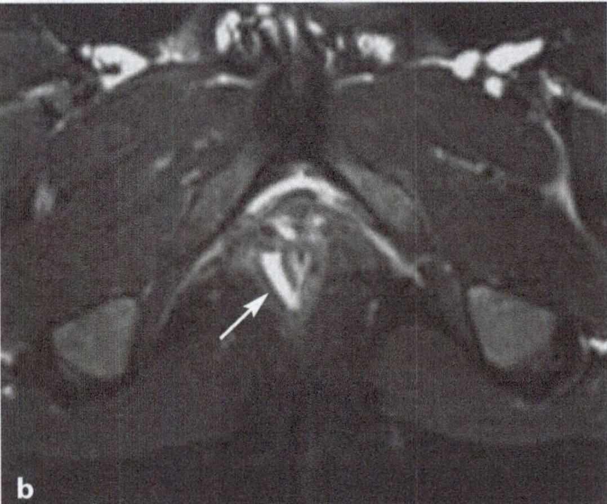

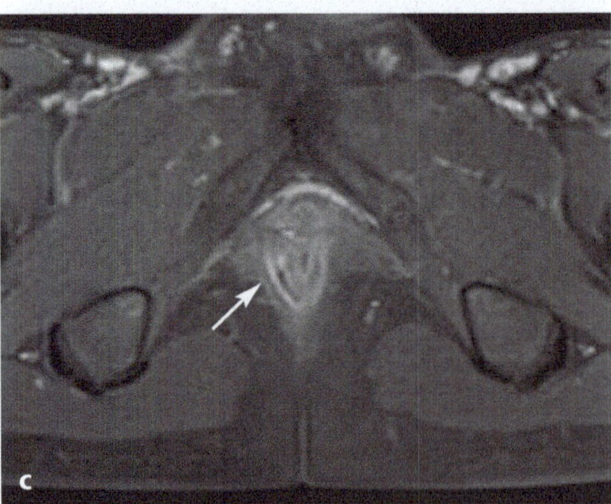

Fig. 20.2 Intersphincteric fistula, grade 1 according to St James University Hospital (SJUH) classification (Parks type I). **a** Axial high-resolution T2-weighted turbo spin echo image shows a linear hyperintensity in the intersphincteric right space (*arrow*). **b** On the axial high-resolution T2-weighted fat-suppressed image, the focal hyperintensity in the intersphincteric left space is more clearly detected (*arrow*). **c** The axial T1-weighted turbo spin echo fat-suppressed image acquired after Gd IV injection shows an enhancing focal lesion corresponding to an intersphincteric fistula. **d** Coronal T2-weighted fat-suppressed image showing the intersphincteric tract (*arrow*). **e** Scheme of a grade 1 fistula according to the SJUH classification (Parks type I) (cont. →)

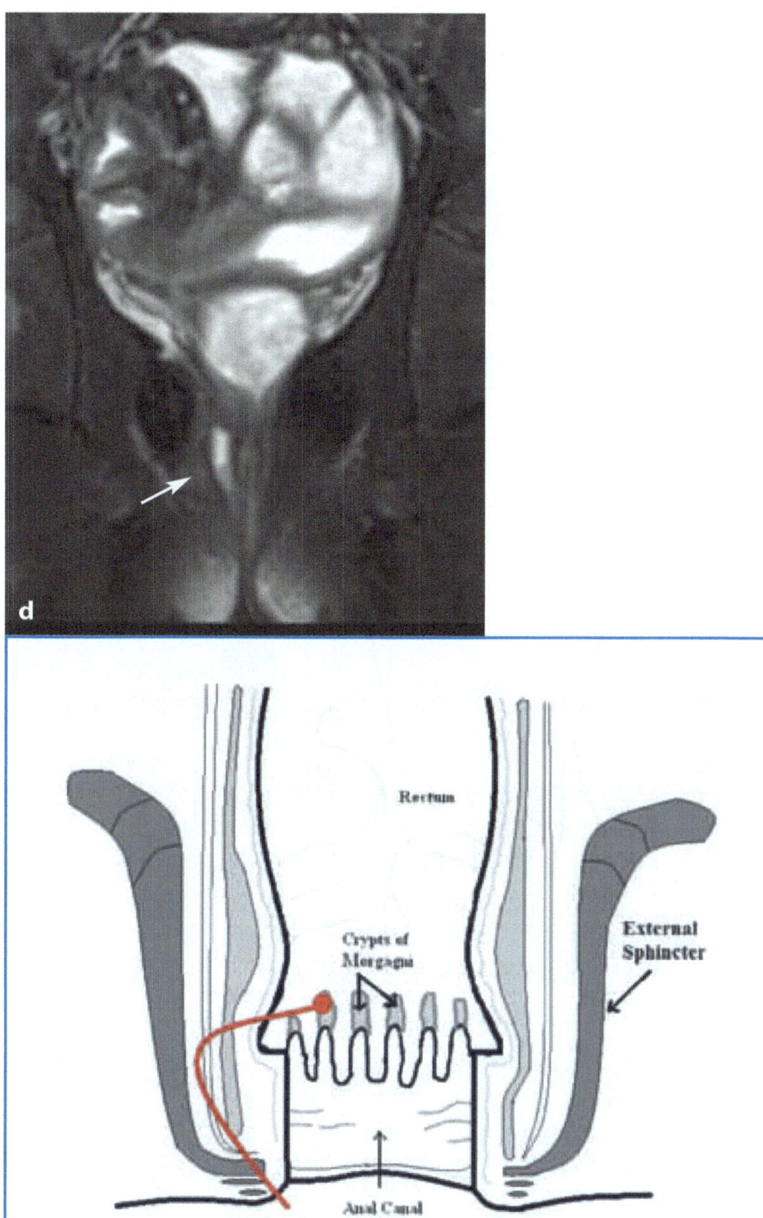

Fig. 20.2 (continued)

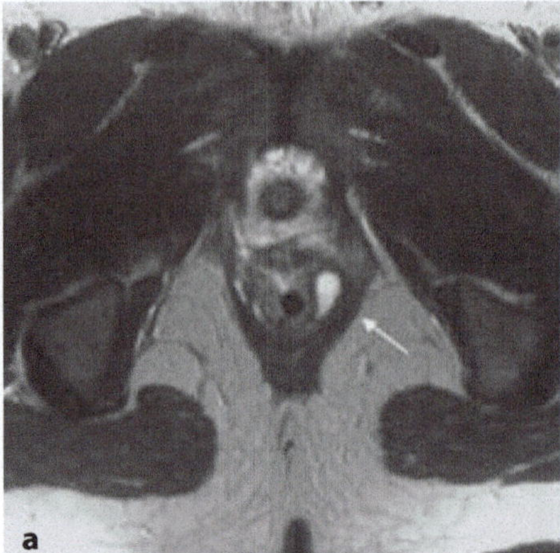

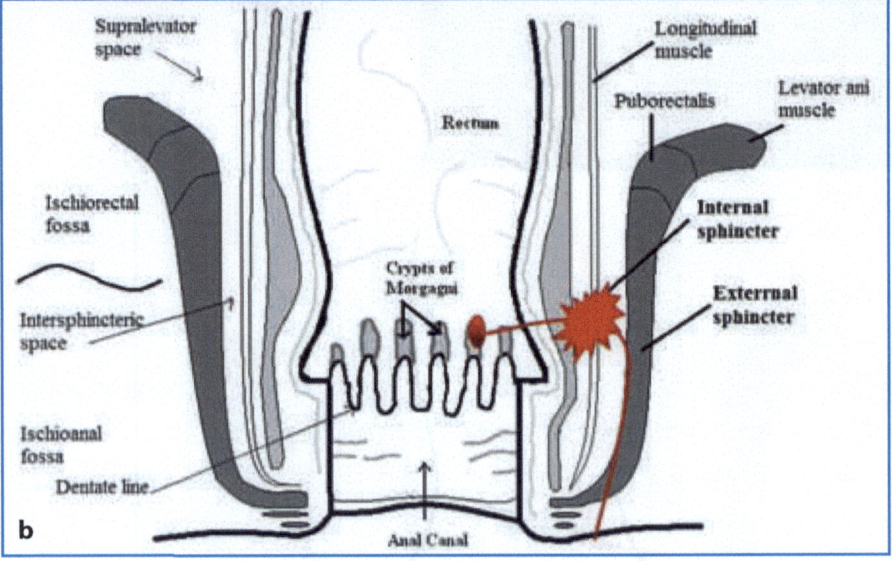

Fig. 20.3 Intersphincteric fistula with a small intersphincteric abscess, grade 2 according to St James University Hospital (SJUH) classification (Parks type I). **a** Axial high-resolution T2 sequence showing a thin intersphincteric posterior horseshoe tract, associated to a small left intersphincteric abscess at three o'clock (*arrow*). **b** Scheme of a grade 2 fistula according to the SJUH classification (Parks type I)

20.2 Radiological and Clinical Classification of Perianal Fistulas

Since relevant MRI findings are not included in the Parks classification, an MRI-based classification was proposed that relates the Parks surgical classification to anatomic MRI findings in the axial and coronal planes. The St James' University Hospital classification was proposed by radiologists on the basis of imaging findings and does not represent an official surgical reference. In fact, in the evaluation of perianal fistulas radiologists are expected to be descriptive and accurate in their reports, as the details of the information they provide will be essential in future decisions regarding medical or surgical treatment [7, 8].

Unlike the Parks classification, that of St James takes into consideration the secondary tracts and abscesses, as well as the primary tract [9]. Since secondary tracts can be missed by clinical examination, preoperative MRI has emerged to better define the fistula anatomy, select the surgical approach, and thereby avoid recurrence [10-13]. All perianal fistulas are divided into five subtypes (Table 20.2). Suprasphincteric and extrasphincteric fistulas are placed in the same category as grade V (supralevator disease). A *grade 1 fistula* is a simple linear intersphincteric fistula (Fig. 20.2) that travels in the intersphincteric space (not disturbing the external sphincter or the ischioanal fossa) and ends at the skin of the perineum or natal cleft. No extensions or abscesses are found in the intersphincteric space or in the ischiorectal and ischioanal fossae. Unlike simple fistulas, a *grade 2 fistula* is intersphincteric, with an abscess or secondary tracts (Fig. 20.3) that are also confined within the intersphincteric space. Secondary tracts of grade 2 fistulas may be of the horseshoe type (lying horizontally and crossing the midline) or they may be on the ipsilateral side of the intersphincteric space. A *grade 3 fistula* is transsphincteric, penetrating both layers of the sphincter complex and directed toward the skin, running through the ischioanal fossa (Fig. 20.4). This type of fistula is of high risk of causing anal incontinence because during surgery the external sphincter must be excised when the tract is opened. In a *grade 4 fistula* (transsphincteric fistula with abscess or secondary tract), the ischioanal fossa harbors an abscess and/or secondary tract, as well as the primary tract (Fig. 20.5). Suprasphincteric and extrasphincteric fistulas are *grade 5* (Figs. 20.6, 20.7).

Table 20.2 MRI classification: St James University Hospital system (from [4])

Grade 0:	Normal aspect
Grade 1:	Simple linear intersphincteric fistula
Grade 2:	Complex intersphincteric fistula with abscess or secondary tract (horseshoe fistula)
Grade 3:	Transsphincteric fistula
Grade 4:	Transsphincteric fistula with abscess or secondary tract within the ischioanal or ischiorectal fossa
Grade 5:	Suprasphincteric and translevator fistulas

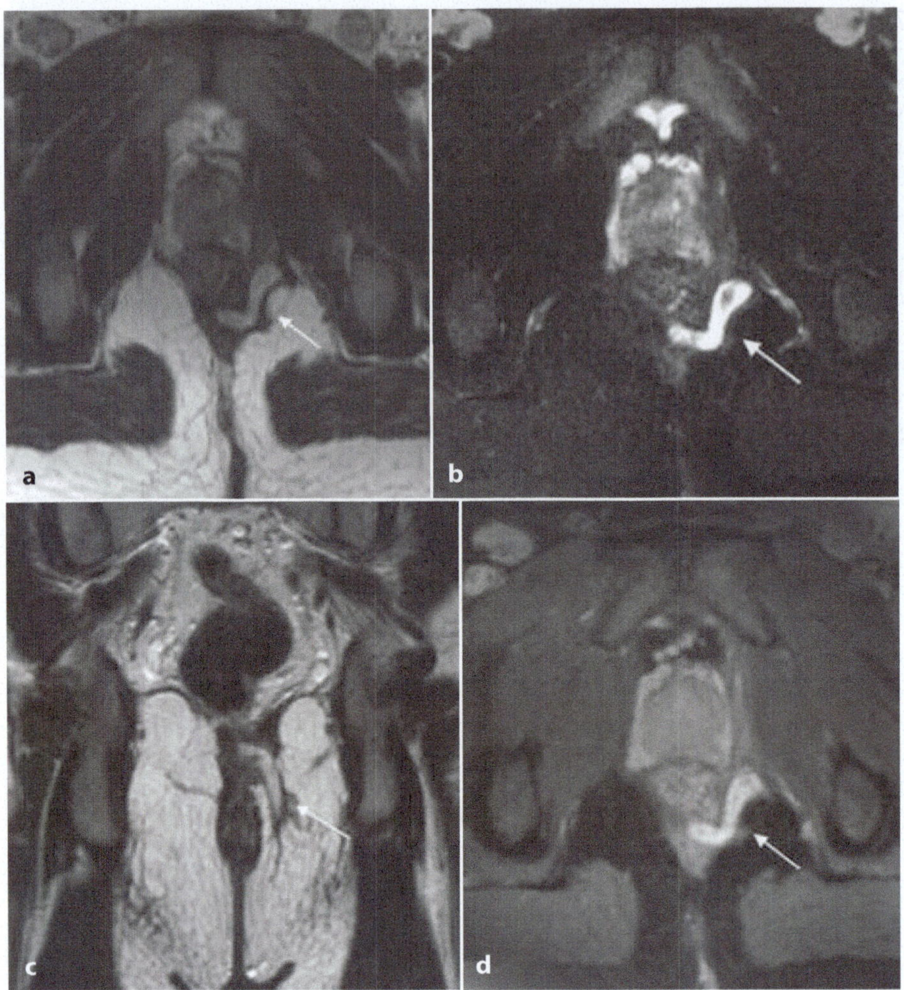

Fig. 20.4 (see next page)

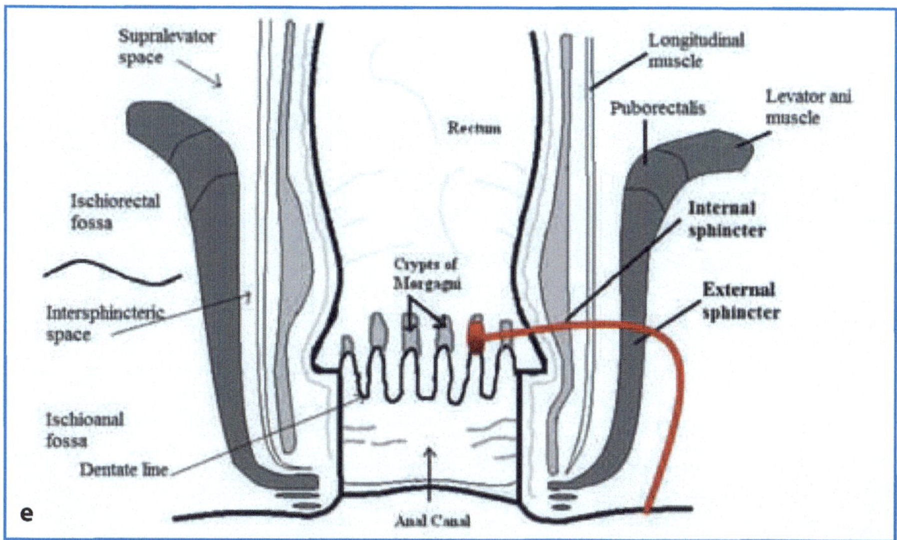

Fig. 20.4 Transsphincteric fistula grade 3 according to the St James University Hospital (SJUH) classification (Parks type II). **a** Axial high-resolution T2 sequence fat-suppressed showing a tubular hyperintense fluid collection (*arrow*) in the posterior anal region (at five-six o'clock) extending through the external sphincter into the ischioanal left fossa. **b** The hyperintense tract filled with fluid is more clearly detected on the axial high-resolution fat-suppressed T2 weighted image, (*arrow*). **c** Coronal high-resolution T2 sequence showing the tubular hyperintense tract extending through the external sphincter into the left ischioanal fossa (*arrow*). **d** Axial T1 turbo spin echo fat-suppressed image acquired after Gd IV injection: in the same area shows an enhancing transsphincteric fistula (*arrow*) (grade 3 SJUH). **e** Grade 3 fistula (*arrow*) according to the SJUH classification (Parks type II)

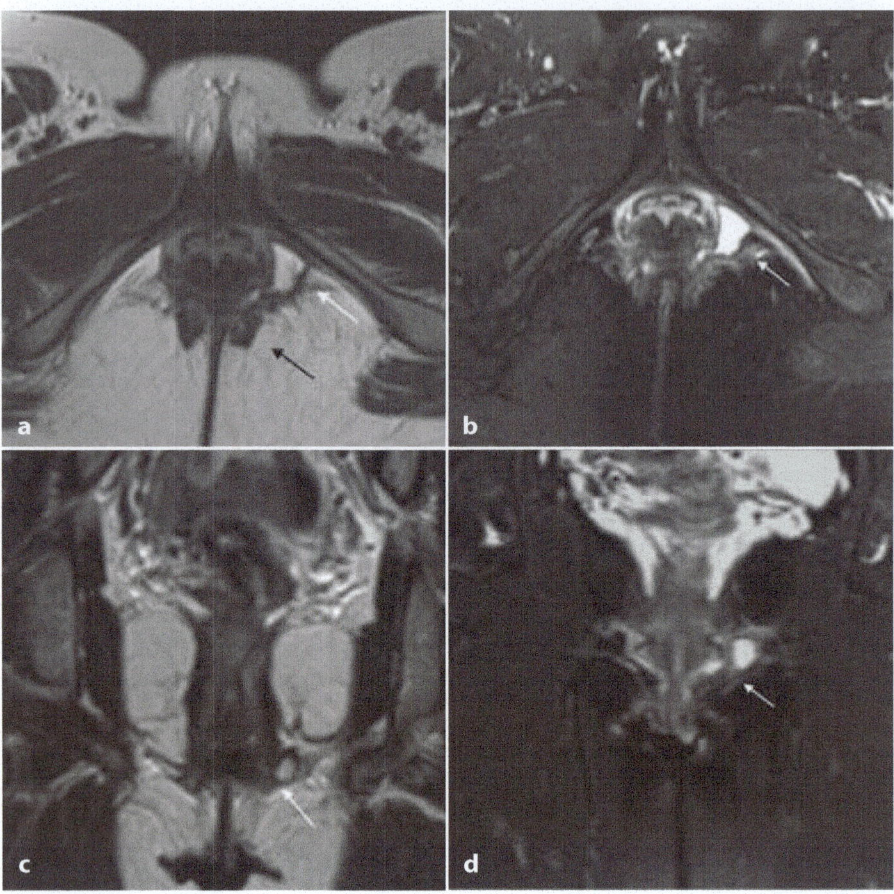

Fig. 20.5 (see next page)

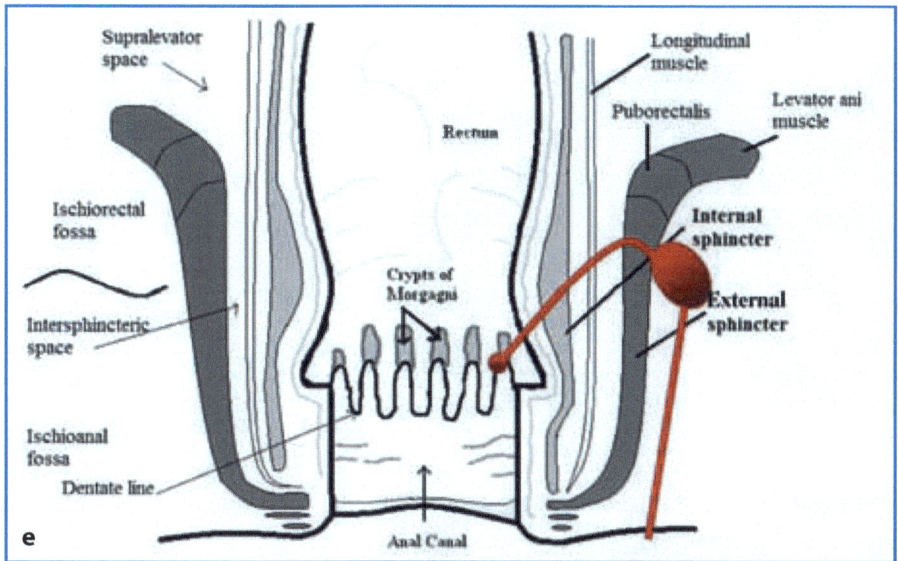

Fig. 20.5 Transsphincteric fistula complicated by an abscess, classified as grade 4 St James University Hospital (SJUH) system (Parks type II). a, b High-resolution T2 weighted plain (**a**) and fat-suppressed (**b**) axial images show a linear transsphincteric hyperintense left fistula (*black arrow*) extending into the ischioanal left fossa and complicated by an abscess (*white arrow*). **c,d** Coronal T2-weighted Hire BEST plain (**c**) and fat-suppressed (**d**) images show a transsphincteric abscess. **e** Scheme of a grade 4 fistula according to the SJUH classification (Parks type II)

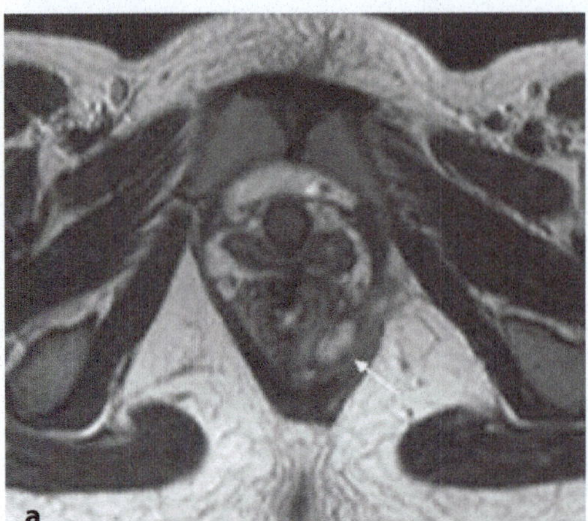

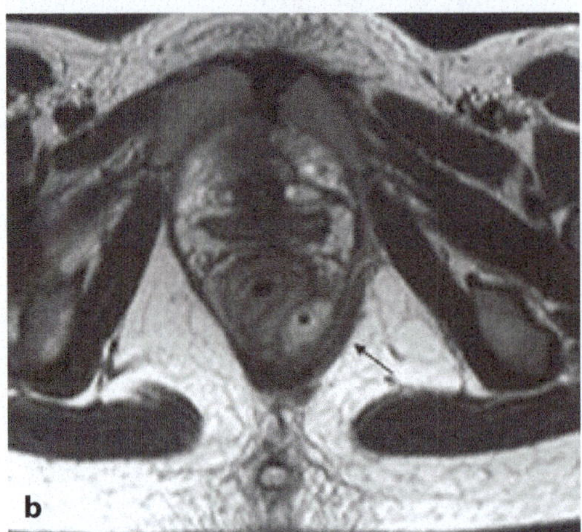

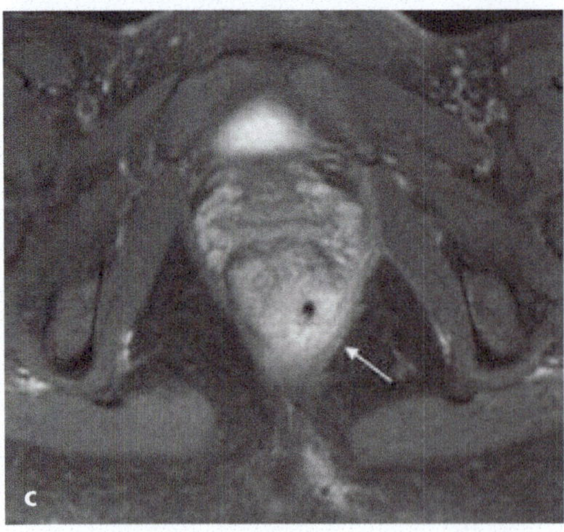

Fig 20.6 (see next page)

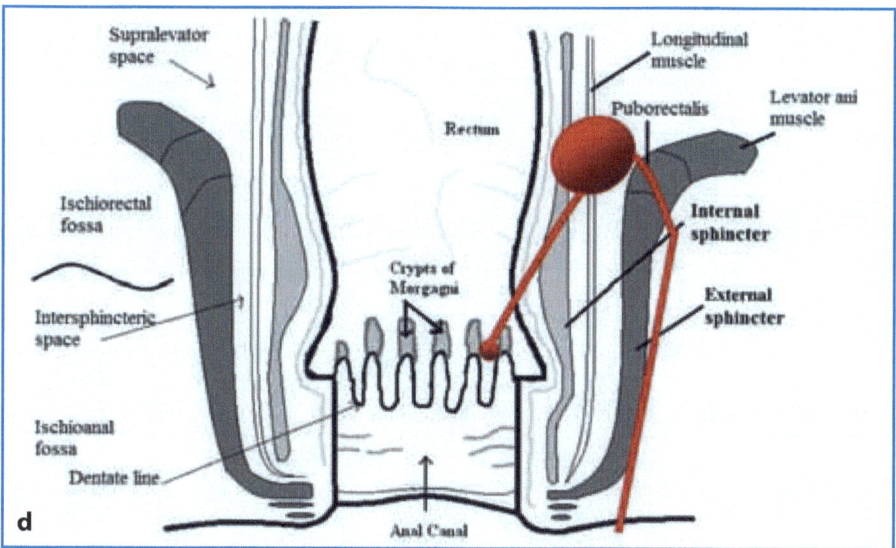

Fig. 20.6 Suprasphincteric fistula with a small abscess, corresponding to grade 5 St James University Hospital (SJUH) classification (Parks type III). **a, b** Axial high-resolution T2 weighted images at different planes. The primary left intersphincteric tract (a) at 4 o'clock (*arrow*) passes above the puborectalis muscle, producing a small pararectal suprasphincteric left abscess (*arrow*) containing a small gas bubble (**b**, **c**). **c** Axial T1-weighted Gd-enhanced image shows the left pararectal supralevator ani abscess. **d** Scheme of a grade 5 fistula according to the SJUH classification (Parks type III)

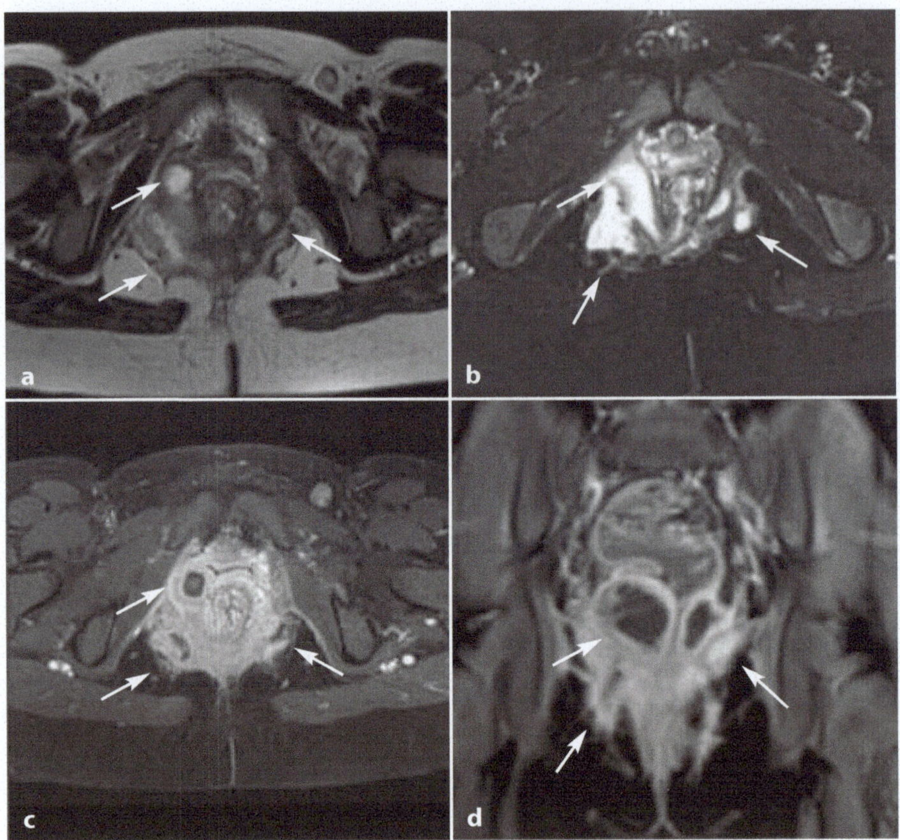

Fig. 20.7 (see next page)

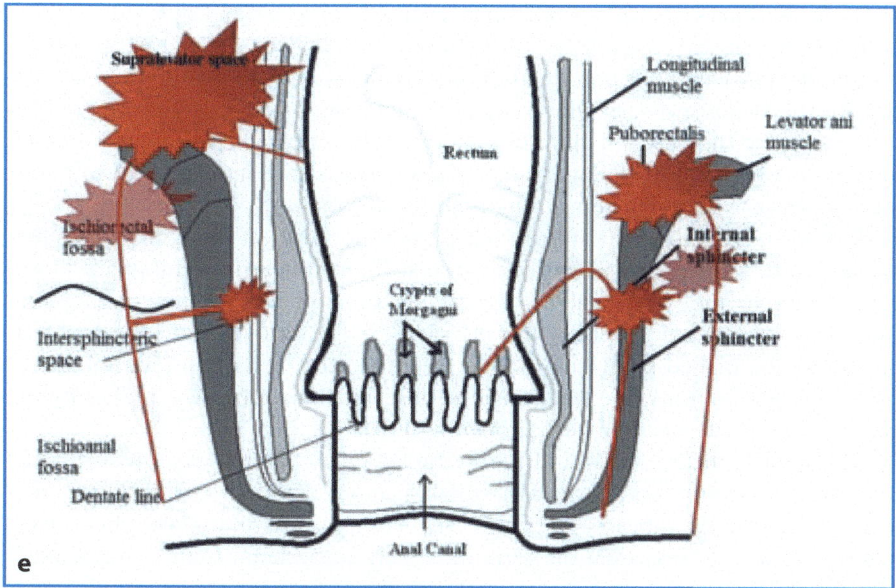

Fig. 20.7 Translevator fistula with multiple abscesses, corresponding to grade 5 of the St James Hospital classification. **a** Axial Hire BEST T2-weighted image shows multiple bilateral abscesses (*arrows*) that extensively involve the levator ani muscle. **b** Axial T2 high-resolution image of multiple translevator abscesses are more clearly detected on fat-suppressed T2 sequences obtained at the same level (*arrows*). **c** Axial T1-weighted Gd-enhanced image showing multiple bilateral translevator abscesses enhancing fluid collections (*arrows*). **d** Coronal T1-weighted Gd-enhanced sequence showing the bilateral translevator abscesses (*arrows*). **e** Schematic representation of multiple bilateral translevator abscesses

As in the Parks classification, supralevator fistulas extend upward through the intersphincteric plane, pass over the top of the levator ani and puborectalis muscle, then descend through the ischiorectal and ischioanal fossae to reach the skin. In translevator disease, the fistulous tract extends directly from its origin in the pelvis to the perineal skin through the ischiorectal and ischioanal fossae, with no involvement of the anal canal. These fistulas are indicative of primary pelvic disease with extension through the levator plate [8, 12].

A small percentage of fistulas (subsphincteric) are left unclassified by the two above-described classification systems. Subsphincteric fistulas are blind tracts lying in the subcutaneous fat tissue, outside the sphincter complex. These blind tracts are generally termed sinuses. They can be detected by MRI and are distinguished from true fistulas, owing to the lack of an internal opening. In these situations, the tract must be described anatomically, including its course and the site of the external opening [13].

Although both the Parks and the St James classification systems are adequate in describing most perianal fistulas, a more detailed description of the disease process has been suggested for complex fistulas. An alternative anatomic-clinical classification pertaining only to perianal fistulas associated with Crohn's disease was proposed by the American Gastroenterology Association (AGA), which classifies these fistulas as *simple* or *complex*. A simple fistula is a superficial, intersphinteric or low transsphincteric fistula that has only one opening and is not associated with an abscess and/or does not connect to an adjacent structure, such as the vagina or bladder. On the contrary, a complex fistula is one that involves more extensively the anal sphincter (i.e., high transsphincteric, extrasphincteric, or suprasphincteric), has multiple openings, exhibits horseshoeing, and is associated with a perianal abscess and/or connected to an adjacent structure, such as the vagina [14]. Other classification systems for fistulas have also been described, including the Montreal classification and the Hughes-Cardiff classification (UFS) [15, 16]. The Montreal system simply differentiates between high and low, whilst the UFS system is based on the presence of ulceration (U), fistula/abscess (F), and stricture (S). The APD classification is the evolution of the Hughes-Cardiff one, based on associated anal conditions (A), proximal intestinal disease (P), and disease activity in anal locations (D) [16].

At present the various classification systems for perianal fistula have yet to be compared in randomized studies.

20.3 Clinical Scoring Systems

Currently, there is no widely accepted and validated clinical scoring system for perianal fistula in Crohn`s disease (CD). The Crohn's disease activity index (CDAI) measures the intestinal and extraintestinal manifestations of CD but it is not highly specific or accurate in the assessment of perianal disease. Instead, the perianal disease activity index (PDAI) and fistula drainage assessment

(FDA) have been proposed to measure fistula activity in clinical trials. The PDAI evaluates five categories affected by fistulas: discharge, pain, restriction of sexual activity, type of perianal disease, and degree of induration. Each category is graded on a 5-point Likert scale, ranging from no symptoms (score of 0) to severe symptoms (score of 4). The maximal PDAI score (on a 5-point scale) is 20 [17], with a higher score indicating more severe disease. The PDAI may, in the coming years, become the perianal disease equivalent of the CDAI, although it has not been fully validated yet [17].

As the FDA is related to the investigator's subjective evaluation, it may be largely variable and for this reason it is not regarded as a potential standard tool with which to evaluate fistula activity nor has it been validated in large studies.

Despite several attempts to provide MRI criteria for the assessment of fistula activity in perianal CD, a widely accepted imaging severity score is still not available. Several MRI classifications of fistula activity have been proposed but their use has been limited to a few clinical trials [18].

In order to provide a more accurate disease index, Van Assche et al. developed an MRI-based score of disease severity for patients with perianal fistulizing CD [19]. In their scoring system, the most important parameter of local inflammatory activity is T2 hyperintensity, whereas gadolinium-enhanced T1-weighted images are not used for perianal fistula assessment. In T2-weighted images, active fistulas and abscesses are visible as hyperintense lesions due to their fluid contents, while scar tissue is hypointense [20, 21]. The other inflammatory parameters are rectal wall thickening and the presence of fluid collections. To date, the system has been a useful tool for the assessment of response to treatment but its validity also remains to be tested in a larger population to determine its full clinical applicability as well as cut-off values of MRI scores for the different stages of disease activity (i.e., remission, mild, moderate, severe).

Conversely, some authors have found that fistulas are more conspicuous on post-contrast images than on T2-weighted ones [22, 23]. On post-contrast T1-weighted images, a marked increase in the signal intensity of inflammatory tissue can be seen due to increased tissue perfusion and vascular permeability [24]. Since local vascularity and permeability increase with the severity of inflammatory disease [25], hypothetically, the post-contrast enhancement of inflammatory tissue reflects the degree of tissue inflammatory activity. Accordingly, contrast-enhanced MRI may be helpful in differentiating active sepsis from fibrosis. However, only a few trials have investigated the relationship between the contrast enhancement of a fistula and clinical disease activity [7]. Spencer et al. were the first to propose the use of dynamic contrast-enhanced MR sequences to assess the presence of perianal fistulas. They had observed that, after contrast, active tracts showed vivid enhancement while the signal of healed tracts was lower [20]. Horsthuis et al. recently suggested dynamic contrast-enhanced MRI as a means of defining perianal disease activity, as an alternative to PDAI, since rapid gadolinium uptake has been shown to correlate with severe disease whereas there is no significant correlation between PDAI and MRI parameters. This observation suggests that PDAI is partly subject to the patient's perception of his or her disease rather than the anatomic and inflammatory substrate [18].

Diffusion-weighted (DW) imaging is another feasible method for evaluating perianal fistula activity, as shown in a recent study by Hori et al. [27]. Their results underline the additional value of DW-MRI compared to fat-suppressed T2-weighted imaging in the diagnosis of anal fistulas, by increasing the confidence level of radiologists, especially regarding patients with risk factors for reactions to intravenous contrast agents. DW-MRI improves the visualization of the external or internal opening of the fistula as well as the visualization of its extent, although this is only true for active ones. In fact, DW imaging has a poorer spatial resolution than spin echo or gradient echo sequences, although the suppressed signal of non-inflamed tissues allows easier detection of the fistula tract. The diagnostic performance of this technique and its utility in a MRI classification system remain to be established by prospective studies on a larger number of patients.

20.4 Value of MRI in the Classification of Perianal Fistulas vs. Clinical and Diagnostic Investigations

Magnetic resonance imaging has emerged as a reliable and accurate technique in the diagnosis of perianal pathology, combining the diagnostic capabilities of several imaging techniques (endoscopic ultrasound, fistulography, and CT) in a single examination [11-14, 26]. Although pelvic CT is able to visualize perianal fistulas, its usefulness in the assessment of perianal disease remains unclear. Due to its limited contrast resolution, CT poorly distinguishes between the similar soft-tissue densities of the anal sphincters and perianal inflammatory streaking. In some cases, the inner opening of the fistula tract is not at all visible on CT imaging. In addition, vascular structures in perirectal fat tissue can be misinterpreted as fistula tracts. CT also lacks accuracy in identifying the levator ani muscle, such that visualization of a supralevator or ischiorectal abscess is very difficult. The advantages of MRI over CT in the staging of perianal disease are numerous [29, 30]. The soft-tissue contrast of MRI is superior to that of CT in the delineation of the anal sphincter complex. Although multislice CT (MSCT) may reconstruct pelvic images on all spatial planes with adequate resolution, MRI can directly image the pelvis in multiple planes without the need for reconstructions [18]. Pelvic MRI more clearly shows the fistula opening in the intestinal wall as well as the surrounding muscle, skin, and visceral layers. It also enables a detailed description of the anatomic relationships of fistulous lesions with respect to the anal sphincters, in addition to the relationships of fistulas or abscesses with the levator ani muscle, according to the Parks classification. However, due to the high spatial resolution of MRI, neural and tiny vascular structures of the perineum, such as the pudendal and lower gluteal arteries, may sometimes be misinterpreted as fistulous tracts.

Fistulography is another important imaging technique used by radiologists to provide surgeons with an accurate preoperative assessment of patients with fistulas-in-ano [12, 31]. In fistulography, the external opening is catheterized with a fine cannula and a water-soluble contrast agent is gently injected to define the fistula tract. Unfortunately, fistulography has two major drawbacks. First, extensions from the primary tract may fail to fill with contrast material if they are plugged with debris, are very remote, or there is excessive contrast material reflux from either the internal or external opening. Second, the sphincter muscles themselves are not directly imaged, which means that the relationships between any tract and the sphincter must be guessed. Furthermore, an inability to visualize the levator plate means that it can be difficult to decide whether an extension has a supralevator or an infralevator location. Similarly, the exact level of the internal opening in the anal canal is often impossible to determine with an accuracy that is high enough to be of value to the surgeon. The net result is that fistulographic findings are both difficult to interpret and unreliable [12, 31].

Most of the comparative studies between MRI and other imaging techniques, and particularly endocavitary ultrasound, generally agree on the superiority of MRI in the staging of complex fistulas [10-14]. Schwartz et al., in a prospective blinded study comparing EUA (exam under anesthesia), MRI, and anal endosonography, demonstrated a diagnostic accuracy of 91%, 87%, and 91% respectively, with 100% accuracy when any of the two methods were combined [32]. In a comparison of anal endosonography with digital rectal evaluation and MRI in 108 patients with primary fistula tracts, the proportion of fistula tracts correctly classified with each modality was: 61% with digital examination, 81% with anal endosonography, and 91% with MRI [33, 34]. In addition, endosonography allowed correct identification of the internal opening in 91% of the patients vs. 97% with MRI. Thus, it was concluded that endosonography with a high-frequency transducer is superior to digital examination in the preoperative classification of perianal fistula. However, while MRI is superior in all respects, endosonography remains a reasonable alternative for identification of the internal opening [33, 35]. Accordingly, the crucial role of MRI in both the preoperative evaluation of perianal fistula and patient outcome is becoming increasingly recognized. The true potential of MRI in the assessment of anal fistulas became evident in a study of 16 patients with cryptoglandular fistulas, comparing MRI findings with the subsequent findings from EUA [34, 35]. The authors concluded that MRI is the most accurate method for determining the presence and course of anal fistulas and that it may help to reduce recurrences due to inaccurate surgical assessment. These conclusions were confirmed in a follow-up study of 35 patients in which MRI assessments were correctly reported in 33 patients (94%), including two in whom EUA failed to identify distant sepsis [36]. In a recent study [39], Schaefer et al. investigated a new MRI protocol, subtraction MR-fistulography, for the detection of fistula-in-ano. This protocol seems to be an important complement to surgical exploration and is especially suitable for investigating complex anal sepsis. In another study [36], in which 56 patients with anal fistulas underwent high-spatial-resolution MRI, this modality was shown to provide important additional information on secondary extensions and recurrent fistulas, particularly in patients with CD. The authors therefore recommended MRI for the preoperative work-up [36, 38]. Finally, the results of MRI, anal endosonography, and clinical examination with the use of evidence-based medicine methods were compared to determine the optimal technique for classifying perianal fistulas. MRI was shown to be optimal for distinguishing complex from simple perianal fistulas, although anal endosonography is superior to clinical examination and may be used if the availability of MRI is limited [8, 33, 37]. Taken together, the results of these studies confirm MRI as the technique of choice in the evaluation of perianal fistulas and associated complications [8].

20.5 Conclusions

Based on its accuracy, non-invasiveness, and lack of ionizing radiation, with only rare contraindications, MRI can be considered as a valuable imaging modality for both the diagnosis and the preoperative classification of anal and perianal fistulas. MRI can detect fistulas both in their early and advanced stages, providing crucial information on the relationships of the fistula with the anal sphincter complex, the levator ani, and the pelvic floor that is not obtained with other imaging modalities (endoscopic ultrasound, fistulography, and CT), which accordingly currently play limited roles in the evaluation of perianal fistulas [29, 12, 30, 31-36].

Based on the advantages of MRI, radiologists can classify perianal fistulas using the St James's University Hospital grading system, which takes into consideration secondary tracts and abscesses, as well as the primary tract. Thus, MRI effectively addressing the appropriate surgical treatment, can decrease the incidence of recurrence and avoid the development of side effects such as fecal incontinence [8].

References

1. Nordgren S, Fasth S, Hulten L et al. (1992) Anal fistulas in Crohn's disease: incidence and outcome of surgical treatment. Int J Colorect Dis 7:214-218
2. Williams JG, Rothenberger DA, Nemer FD et al (1991) Fistula-in-ano in Crohn's disease. Results of aggressive surgical treatment. Dis Colon Rectum 34:378-384
3. Parks AG, Morson BC (1962) Fistula in ano. The pathogenesis of fistula in ano. Proc R Soc Med 55:751-754
4. Lilius HG (1968) Investigation of human foetal anal ducts and intramuscular glands and a clinical study of 150 patients. Acta Chir Scand (Suppl. 383)
5. Milligan FTC, Morgan CN (1934) Surgical anatomy of the anal canal with special reference to ano-rectal fistulae. Lancet 2:1150-1213
6. Parks AG (1969a) The classification of fistula in ano. In Hoferichter J (ed.) Progress in Proctology New York Springer pp:30-35

7. Morris J, Spencer JA, Ambrose NS (2000) MR imaging classification of perianal fistulas and its implications for patient management. Radiographics 20:623–35
8. De Miguel Criado J, García del Salto L, Fraga Rivas P et al (2012) MR Imaging Evaluation of Perianal Fistulas: Spectrum of Imaging Features. Radiographics 32:175-194
9. Al-Khawari HA, Gupta R, Sinan TS et al (2005) Role of magnetic resonance imaging in the assessment of perianal fistulas. Med Princ Pract 14:46–52
10. Spencer JA, Chapple K, Wilson D et al (1998) Outcome after surgery for perianal fistula: predictive value of MR imaging. AJR Am J Roentgenol 171: 403–6.
11. Maccioni F, Colaiacomo MC, Stasolla A et al (2002) Value of MRI performed with phased-array coil in the diagnosis and preoperative classification of perianal and anal fistulas. La Radiologia Medica - Radiol Med 103: 000-000
12. Halligan S, Stoker J (2006) Imaging of fistula in ano. Radiology 239:18–33.
13. Berman L, Israel GM, McCarthy SM et al (2007) Utility of magnetic resonance imaging in anorectal disease. World J Gastroenterol 13:3153–8.
14. Wise PE, Schwartz DA (2006) Management of perianal Crohn's disease. Clin Gastroenterol Hepatol 4:426-30.
15. Satsangi J, Silverberg MS, Vermeire S et al (2006) The Montreal classification of inflammatory bowel disease: controversies, consensus, and implications. Gut. Consensus Development Conference. 55(6):749-53
16. Hughes LE (1992) Clinical classification of perianal Crohn's disease. Dis Colon Rectum. 35:928–932
17. Irvine EJ (1995) Usual therapy improves perianal Crohn disease as measured by New Disease Activity index. Mc Master IBD Study Group. J Clin Gastroenterol 20: 27-32
18. Horsthuis K, Lavini C, Bipat S et al (2009) Perianal Crohn disease: evaluation of dynamic contrast-enhanced MR imaging as an indicator of disease activity. Radiology 251(2):380-7
19. Van Assche G, Vanbeckevoort D, Bielen D et al (2003) Magnetic resonance imaging of the effects of infliximab on perianal fistulizing Crohn's disease. Am J Gastroenterol 98:332–9
20. Spencer JA, Ward J, Beckingham IJ et al (1996) Dynamic contrast-enhanced MR imaging of perianal fistulas. AJR 167:735–41
21. Tissot O, Bodnar D, Henry L et al (1996) Ano-perineal fistula in MRI. Contribution of T2 weighted sequences. Article in French J Radiol 77:253–60.
22. Schmidt S, Chevallier P, Bessoud B et al (2007) Diagnostic performance of MRI for detection of intestinal fistulas in patients with complicated inflammatory bowel conditions. Eur Radiol 17:2957–63
23. Semelka RC, Hricak H, Kim B et al (1997) Pelvic fistulas: appearances on MR images. Abdom Imaging 22:91–5
24. Weinmann HJ, Brasch RC, Press WR et al (1984) Characteristics of gadolinium-DTPA complex: a potential NMR contrast agent. AJR Am J Roentgenol 142:619–24
25. Brahme F, Lindstrom C (1970) A comparative radiographic and pathological study of intestinal vaso-architecture in Crohn's disease and in ulcerative colitis. Gut 11:928–40
26. Van Dijke CF, Peterfry CG, Brasch RC et al (1999) MR imaging of the arthritic rabbit knee joint using albumin (Gd-DTPA) 30 with correlation to histopathology. Magn Reson Imaging 17:237–45
27. Hori M, Oto A, Orrin S et al (2009) Diffusion-weighted MRI: a new tool for the diagnosis of fistula in ano. J Magn Reson Imaging 30:1021–1026
28. Sun MR, Smith MP, Kane RA (2008) Current techniques in imaging of fistula in ano: three-dimensional endoanal ultrasound and magnetic resonance imaging. Semin Ultrasound CT MR 29:454–71
29. Furukawa A, Saotome T, Yamasaki M et al (2004) Cross-sectional imaging in Crohn disease. Radiographics 24:689–702
30. Koelbel G, Schmiedl U et al (1989) Diagnosis of fistulae and Sinus Tract in Patients with Crohn Disease: Value of MR Imaging. AJR 152: 999-1003

31. Kuijpers HC, Schulpen T (1985) Fistulography for fistula-in-ano: is it useful? Dis Colon Rectum 28:103–104
32. Schwartz DA, Wiersema MJ, Dudiak KM et al (2001) A comparison of endoscopic ultrasound,magnetic resonance imaging, and exam under anesthesia for evaluation of Crohn's perianal fistulas. Gastroenterology 121:1064–1072
33. Buchanan GN, Halligan S, Bartram CI et al (2004) Clinical examination, endosonography, and MR imaging in preoperative assessment of fistula in ano: comparison with outcome-based reference standard. Radiology 233(3):674–681
34. Lunniss PJ, Armstrong P, Barker PG et al (1992) Magnetic resonance imaging of anal fistulae. Lancet 340(8816):394–396.
35. Lunniss PJ, Barker PG, Sultan AH et al (1994) Magnetic resonance imaging of fistula-in-ano. Dis Colon Rectum 37(7):708–718
36. Beets-Tan RG, Beets GL, van der Hoop AG et al (2001) Preoperative MR imaging of anal fistulas: does it really help the surgeon? Radiology 218 (1):75–84
37. Sahni VA, Ahmad R, Burling D (2008) Which method is best for imaging of perianal fistula? Abdom Imaging 33(1):26–30
38. Ziech M, Felt-Bersma R, Stoker J (2009) Imaging of perianal fistulas. Clin Gastroenterol Hepatol 7 (10):1037–1045
39. Schaefer O, Lohrmann C, Langer M (2004) Assessment of anal fistulas with high-resolution subtraction MR-fistulography: comparison with surgical findings. J Magn Reson Imaging 19 (1):91-8

Diagnostic Accuracy of MRI in Perianal Crohn's Disease

21

Chiara Villa

In the last decades, the role of magnetic resonance imaging (MRI) in the evaluation of perianal disease has been investigated and its accuracy in the diagnosis of anal fistulas is now well established, especially in patients with Crohn's disease (CD). Today, MRI is considered the gold standard for the imaging of anal fistulas [1, 2].

In 1989, Koelbel et al. were the first to study the potential role of MRI in the evaluation of sinus tracts and fistulas associated with CD, comparing the results with those of contrast-enhanced CT, barium studies, endoscopy, and sonography. The authors showed that due to its multiplanarity, high soft-tissue contrast resolution, and lack of ionizing radiation, MRI was more accurate in depicting the exact extension of the fistula [3].

Barker et al. confirmed the high degree of accuracy of MRI in demonstrating the topography of anal fistulas, reporting concordance rates between MRI and surgical findings of 86% for the presence and course of the primary tract, 91% for the presence and site of secondary extensions or abscesses, and 97% for the presence of horseshoeing [4].

Beets-Tan et al. reported that, compared with surgical data, the sensitivity and specificity of MRI in the detection of the primary tract of the fistula were, respectively, 100% and 86%. In the detection of abscesses and horseshoe fistulas the rates were 96% and 97%, and 100% and 100%, respectively, while in the detection of internal openings rates of 96% and 90%, respectively, were reported [5].

More recently, the 2003 position paper from the American Gastroenterological Association (AGA) recommended the use of MRI in the preoperative assessment of perianal fistulas, and in 2006 the European Crohn's and Colitis

C. Villa (✉)
Radiology Department, Luigi Sacco University Hospital
Milan, Italy
e-mail: chiara.villa@hotmail.it

M.Tonolini and G. Maconi (eds.), *Imaging of Perianal Inflammatory Diseases*,
DOI: 10.1007/978-88-470-2847-0_21, © Springer-Verlag Italia 2013

Organization (ECCO) considered the use of MRI mandatory in the evaluation of the response to medical or surgical treatment of perianal fistulas, either as the sole imaging modality or in combination with anorectal endoscopic ultrasonography (EUS) or clinical examination under anesthesia (EUA) [6, 7].

In any known complex fistula, including all recurrent and Crohn's-related fistulas, MRI is now considered the examination of choice as it is able to detect the presence of sepsis outside the sphincter, to show the relationship of the fistula to the sphincter and levator muscles, and to distinguish active sepsis from fibrosis [8, 9]. Moreover, recent studies demonstrated the reliability and usefulness of MRI in monitoring fistula healing during infliximab therapy, based on the ability of MRI to detect clinically silent sepsis in the internal fistula tract, despite closure of the draining external orifices [10-15].

We carried out a study evaluating the accuracy of MRI and transperineal ultrasound in the assessment of perianal Crohn's disease among 51 patients with CD, considering as reference standard the combined surgical examination and imaging findings. In this series of 65 fistulas (9 anovaginal and 56 perianal, classified according to the Parks criteria) and 17 abscesses were diagnosed. Perianal CD was staged according to the AGA criteria as simple (39.2% of patients) and complex (60.8% of patients). MRI diagnosed one or more fistulas in 41 patients (per-patient sensitivity 87.2%), detecting 51 out of 56 perianal fistulas (per-lesion sensitivity 91.1%) and four out of nine anovaginal fistulas (per-lesion sensitivity 44.4%). MRI correctly classified 50 (positive predictive value 98%) perianal fistulas according to the Parks criteria and four (positive predictive value 100%) anovaginal tracts. All 17 (sensitivity 100%) abscesses were properly identified. Moreover, MRI evaluation of simple or complex perianal disease led to an exact diagnosis in 47 (92.1%) cases.

MRI was also demonstrated to be a reliable diagnostic tool, showing a sensitivity (87.2%) and positive predictive values (98%) in agreement with previous literature data [5].

Anovaginal fistulas were neither detected nor correctly classified by MRI (sensitivity < 50%) because of their location in a small, virtually adipose space between the anal canal and the vagina that is undetectable on MR scans acquired with surface phased array coils, as previously reported [16]. Conversely, all perianal abscesses, mostly located in the ischioanal fossa or above the levator ani muscle, were detected with MRI, given the large field of view achieved with surface coils and the high contrast resolution provided by fat-suppressed and contrast-enhanced sequences.

References

1. Morris J, Spencer JA, Ambrose NS (2000) MR imaging classification of perianal fistulas and its implications for patients management. Radiographics 20:623-637
2. Halligan S, Stoker J (2006) Imaging of fistula in ano. Radiology 239:18-33
3. Koelbel G, Schmiedl U, Majer MC et al (1989) Diagnosis of fistulae and sinus tracts in patients with Crohn disease: value of MR imaging. AJR 152:999-1003

4. Barker PG, Lunniss PJ, Armstrong P et al (1994) Magnetic resonance imaging of fistula-in-ano: technique, interpretation and accuracy. Clinical Radiology 49:7-13
5. Beets-Tan RG, Beets GL, van der Hoop AG et al (2001) Preoperative MR imaging of anal fistulas: does it really help the surgeon? Radiology 218:75-84
6. Sandborn WJ, Fazio VW, Feagan BG, Hanauer SB. American Gastroenterological Association Clinical Practice Committee (2003) AGA technical review on perianal Crohn's disease. Gastroenterology 125:1508-1530
7. Caprilli R, Gassull MA, Escher JC et al (2006) European evidence based consensus on the diagnosis and management of Crohn's disease: special situations. Gut 55 (Suppl 1):i36-i58
8. Bartram C, Buchanan G (2003) Imaging anal fistula. Radiol Clin N Am 41:443-457
9. Sahni VA, Ahmad R, Burling D (2008) Which method is best for imaging of perianal fistula? Abdom Imaging 33:26-30
10. Bell SJ, Halligan S, Windsor AC et al (2003) Response of fistulasing Crohn's disease to infliximab treatment assessed by magnetic resonance imaging. Aliment Pharmacol Ther 17: 387-93
11. Van Assche G, Vanbeckevoort D, Bielen D et al (2003) Magnetic resonance imaging of the effects of infliximab on perianal fistulizing Crohn's disease. Am J Gastroenterol 98:332-339
12 Ng SC, Plamondon S, Gupta A et al (2009) Prospective evaluation of anti-tumor necrosis factor therapy guided by magnetic resonance imaging for Crohn's perineal fistulas. Am J Gastroenterol 104:2973-2986
13. Schwarts DA (2009) Imaging and the treatment of Crohn's perianal fistulas: to see is to believe. Am J Gastroenterol 104: 2987-2989
14. Savoye-Collet C, Savoye G, Koning E (2010) Fistulizing perianal Crohn's disease: contrast-enhanced magnetic resonance imaging assessment at one year on maintenance anti-TNF-alpha therapy. Inflamm Bowel Dis 17(8):1751-1758
15. Karmiris K, Bielen D, Vanbeckevoort D et al (2011) Long-term monitoring of infliximab therapy for perianal fistulizing Crohn's disease by using magnetic resonance imaging. Clin Gastroenterol Hepatol. 9:130-136
16. Dwarkasing S, Hussain SM, Hop WCJ et al (2004) Anovaginal fistulas: evaluation with endoanal MR imaging. Radiology 231:123-128

Post-surgical Findings and Post-treatment MRI Follow-Up

22

Massimo Tonolini

22.1 Postoperative MRI Evaluation

Although CT is most commonly performed to image or otherwise rule out acute complications during the early postoperative period following abdomino-pelvic surgery, MRI represents the most valuable modality in the follow-up of procedures involving the anorectal region, particularly to investigate new or recurrent symptoms. Precise knowledge of the surgical history and procedure details is important, since the imaging goal is to document the normal postoperative anatomy, identify septic complications, assess treatment results, and evaluate possible recurrence [1, 2].

Fistulotomy of superficial and simple intersphincteric fistulas is usually not identifiable at MRI [1]. After successful surgical fistulectomy, the treated tract appears with a low signal intensity corresponding to its fibrous walls, best perceptible without fat suppression. The absence of contrast enhancement after intravenous gadolinium should be the rule for healed, non-inflamed tracts after surgery (Fig. 22.1). As more extensively discussed in the chapter on MRI artifacts and pitfalls, persistently high T2-weighted signal intensity and positive contrast enhancement are sometimes observed long after surgery or following therapy-induced clinical remission, probably reflecting unreliable imaging differentiation between persistently active sepsis and healing granulation tissue [1].

Complex perianal inflammatory disease is commonly treated with seton placement, often before or during medical therapy; the band is tied through the fistulous tract to keep it open and draining and may be left in place for months.

M. Tonolini (✉)
Radiology Department, Luigi Sacco University Hospital
Milan, Italy
e-mail: mtonolini@sirm.org

M.Tonolini and G. Maconi (eds.), *Imaging of Perianal Inflammatory Diseases*,
DOI: 10.1007/978-88-470-2847-0_22, © Springer-Verlag Italia 2013

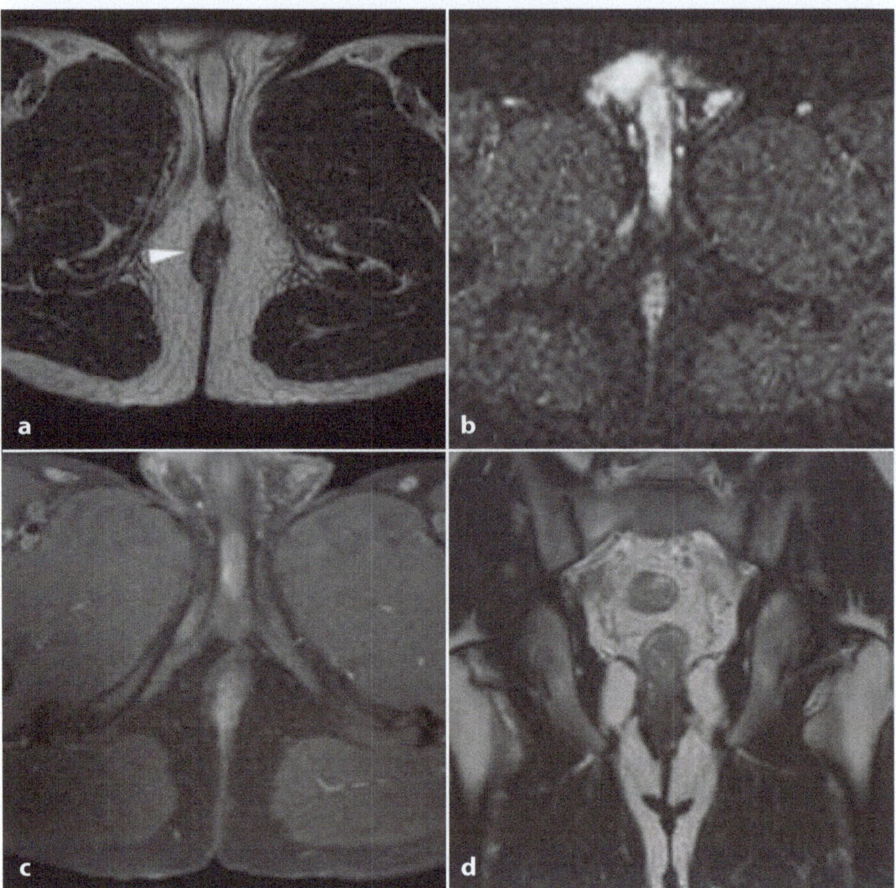

Fig. 22.1 A 56-year-old male patient with Crohn's disease. After surgical fistulectomy in the previous site of a simple transsphincteric fistula, the anal canal shows subtle right-sided hypointense irregularity (arrowhead) on the axial T2-weighted image (**a**) without hyperintense signal on the axial STIR image (**b**) nor abnormal enhancement on the corresponding post-contrast axial fat-suppressed (**c**) and coronal (**d**) T1-weighted images

At MRI, setons appear as thin tubular structures with low signal intensity on all sequences; they are best identified within a fluid-containing T2-hyperintense fistulous tract or abscess collection (Fig. 22.2). An alternative surgical option is the positioning of a draining large-caliber Foley catheter [3].

Owing to its precise reproducibility, with high contrast and spatial resolution (Figs. 22.3, 22.4), MRI is the imaging modality of choice to document postoperative appearances, even after more complex surgical procedures, including extensive resection, omentoplasty, and fasciocutaneous flaps, and to investigate suspected complications such as leakages and abscess collections [1, 2].

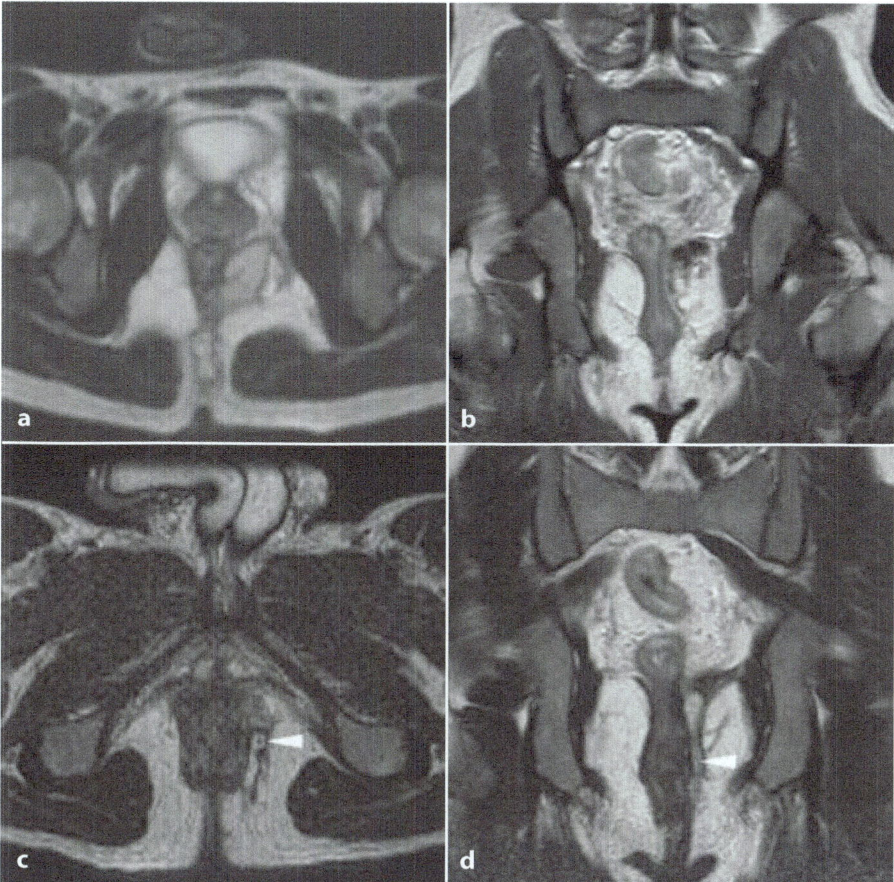

Fig. 22.2 A 32-year-old male patient with Crohn's disease. Initial MRI including axial T2-weighted (**a**) and contrast-enhanced coronal T1-weighted (**b**) images shows a large abscess collection occupying the left levator ani muscle. After treatment via a surgical approach, follow-up MRI consisting of axial (**c**) and coronal (**d**) T2-weighted images shows abscess reduction with the seton (*arrowheads*) in place

22.2 MRI Follow-Up During and After Infliximab Therapy

Treatment with the anti-tumor necrosis factor (anti-TNF) antibody infliximab has been shown to effectively achieve rapid closure of anal fistulas, although its mechanism of action is still poorly understood. Fistula healing is undoubtedly a refractory and slow process although its rate, extent, and duration are under investigation. After induction therapy, the clinical response is often short and maintenance therapy at scheduled intervals is usually required [4-8].

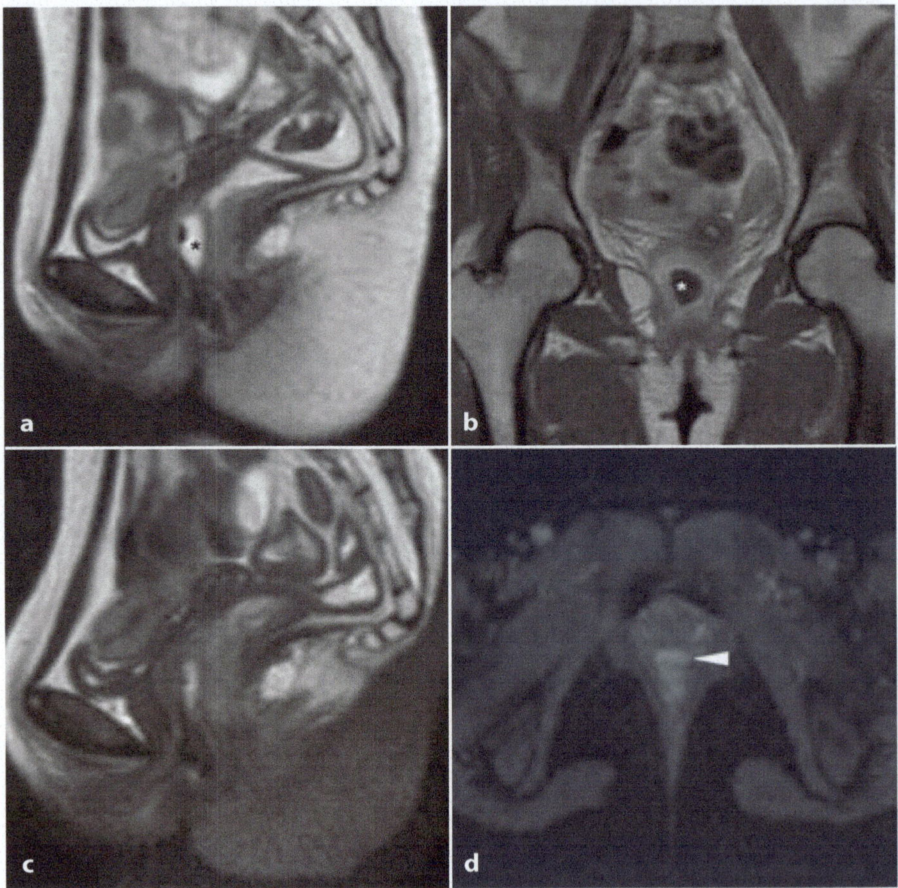

Fig. 22.3 A 27-year-old female patient with Crohn's disease. Initial MRI including sagittal T2-weighted (**a**) and post-contrast coronal T1-weighted (**b**) images detects a large abscess occupying the anovaginal septum (*). After surgical drainage, repeated MRI (**c**, **d**) shows significant reduction, evidenced by the collapsed abscess walls (*arrowheads*)

Preliminary studies have suggested that the cessation of drainage from external orifices does not accurately reflect the true condition of the fistulous tract, since fistulas may persist despite healing of the external openings, leading to abscess formation that may become clinically evident after treatment [3, 6, 9, 10]. The ability of MRI to detect residual active inflammation even with closed orifices makes it particularly suited for the non-invasive assessment of the results of infliximab therapy [10].

The recent ECCO (European Crohn's and Colitis Organization) guidelines recognized the need for pre-treatment imaging and thus recommended MRI or

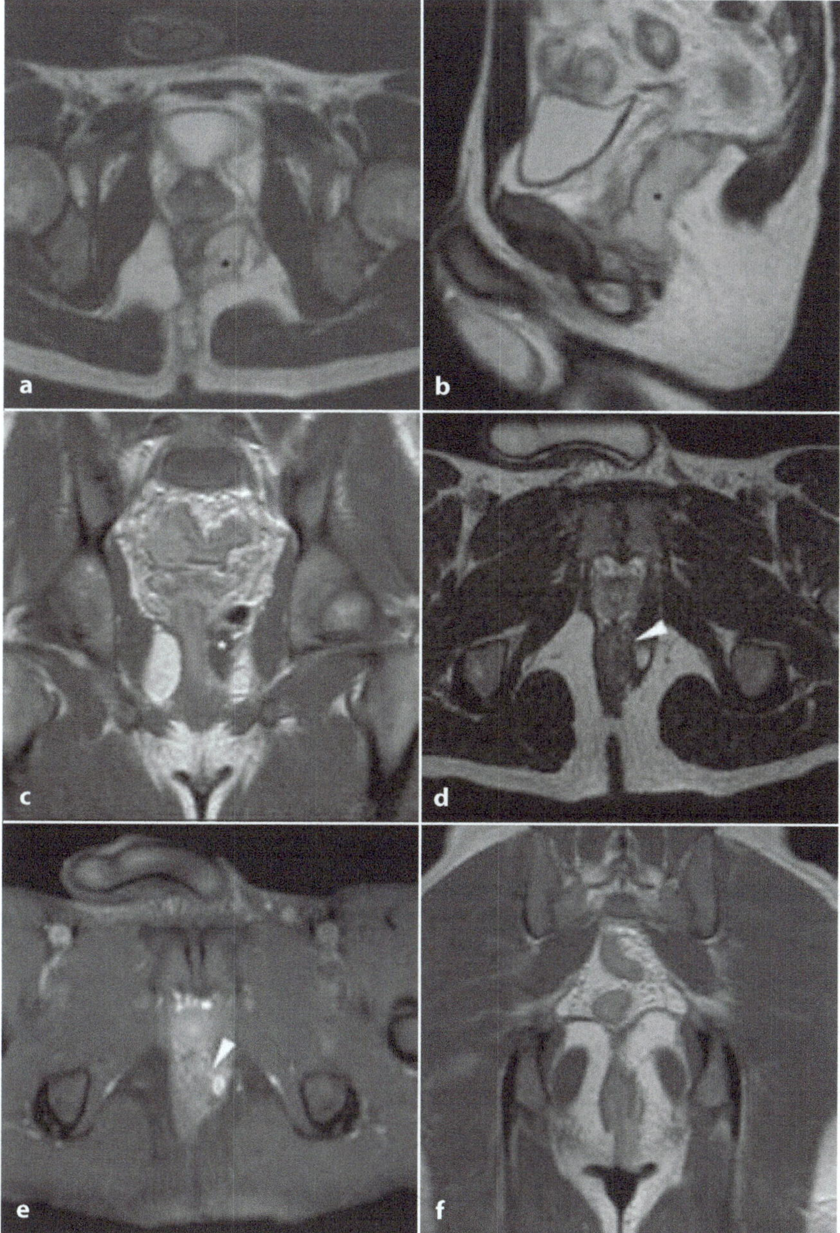

Fig. 22.4 A 25-year-old male patient with Crohn's disease. Initial MRI (**a-c**) showed a large abscess with mixed air and fluid content, extensively involving the left ischioanal fossa and levator ani muscle (*). Complementary transperineal ultrasound revealed the presence of a posterior extrasphinteric fistula. Following seton placement and medical therapy with azathioprine plus infliximab, MRI at one-year follow-up (**d-f**) evidenced a significant reduction of the abscess and a normalization of the levator ani muscle (**f**). The left-sided transsphinteric fistula became visible (*arrowheads* in **d** and **e**) in association with a very small residual ischioanal abscess

endoanal ultrasound for all fistulas under consideration for medical and/or surgical treatment [11].

In 2003, Van Assche et al. published a MRI-based severity score for perianal Crohn's disease that takes into account the anatomical extension of the fistulous tracts along with their T2-hyperintensity in areas of inflammation, the presence of abscess collections, and rectal wall involvement (Table 22.1). Although this scoring system has been validated in the pretherapeutic setting, is easily reproducible, and useful in clinical trials, it notably lacks key information obtainable from MRI, since it does not consider inflammatory activity that is well detected by contrast enhancement [10].

Baseline MRI examinations evaluated prior to infliximab therapy should be carefully analyzed for evidence of clinically occult purulent collections, since their presence may predispose the patient to abscess development during biologic therapy. Anti-TNF drugs are contraindicated in the presence of an abscess [12]; instead, these patients should be referred for drainage or other surgical treatment before infliximab is started [6, 10].

Complex inflammatory disease at baseline is reportedly associated with a worse outcome after medical therapy. Conversely, other investigators have not identified the initial MRI features that reliably predict fistula healing and clinical remission after infliximab treatment [13, 14].

Table 22.1 MRI-based severity score for perianal Crohn's disease (from [10])

Parameter	Score
Number of fistula tracts	
None	0
Single, unbranched	1
Single, branched	2
Multiple	3
Location	
Extra- or intersphincteric	1
Transsphincteric	2
Suprasphincteric	3
Extension	
Infralevator	1
Supralevator	2
Hyperintensity on T2-weighted images	
Absent	0
Mild	4
Pronounced	8
Collections (cavities > 3 mm in diameter)	
Absent	0
Present	4
Rectal wall involvement	
Normal	0
Thickened	2

In most published trials, therapeutic response has been clinically judged by assessing the drainage of external fistulous openings under gentle compression. However, this simple criterion is not only very limited, but it is also inappropriate to correctly assess response and therapy outcome [3, 7-9]. There is mounting evidence supporting the use of MRI in monitoring infliximab therapy in order to detect residual infection, despite clinical findings suggesting remission; the goal is to identify those patients who require prolonged therapy. Initial experiences proposed a follow-up MRI study at least one month after the last infliximab infusion [6, 10]. Paired baseline and post-treatment MRI acquisitions are reviewed, preferentially by the same experienced radiologist (Fig. 22.4). Response may be rated as resolved, better, unchanged, or worsened. A disappearance or reduction in the number of fistulas and/or draining cavities indicates improvement, whereas deterioration is defined by an increase in the number and size of fistulas and cavities or by the development of new lesions [4, 6]. Alternatively, the severity of perianal Crohn's disease may be assessed semi-quantitatively before and after infliximab administration according to the above-cited scoring system of Van Assche et al. [10] (Table 22.1).

Following infliximab therapy, radiological resolution of perianal inflammation at MRI is substantially variable and consistently slower than clinical healing. Complete ("deep") fistula healing was observed in 20%, 28%, and 30% of the examined patients after 6, 12, and 18 months, respectively, even though clinical remission with fistula closure was achieved in half of cases [4]. The persistence of fistulous tracts with high T2-weighted signal intensity and positive contrast enhancement despite the cessation of external drainage is a frequent occurrence and may be related to incomplete histological healing or to the difficult differentiation between residual active sepsis and healing granulation tissue [6]. Importantly, once radiological resolution has been achieved, persistent clinical remission is expected even after infliximab treatment is discontinued. Therefore, complete fistula healing at MRI has been suggested as a useful indicator for therapy termination [4].

The first long-term results of the MRI follow-up of patients with medically treated perianal inflammatory disease were recently reported in the literature [8, 14]. After one year of maintenance therapy, significant improvements in the inflammatory scores (mainly due to the disappearance of abscesses) and decreases in the T2-hyperintense signals were consistently observed in patients with clinical benefit, including response and remission. According to Savoye-Collet et al. [8], disappearance of the fluid-like T2 hyperintense signal of fistulas indicates clinical remission, with a sensitivity, specificity, and positive and negative predictive values of 71.4%, 92.3%, 83.3%, and 85.7%, respectively, reported in their study. A less frequent occurrence (30% of patients) and, as noted above, not included in the scoring system by Van Assche et al. [10], is the complete loss of contrast enhancement; however, this is highly associated with clinical remission (sensitivity, specificity, positive and negative predictive values of 85.7%, 100%, 100%, and 92.8%, respectively). Based on these data, a progressive, multiphase healing process of treated perianal fistulas has been suggested in which an initial decrease and the subsequent cessation of pus production are followed by late repair [8].

Another very recent study reported significant improvement in terms of activity scores and a reduction in the number and inflammatory components of fistulas during maintenance infliximab treatment, both at short-term vs. baseline MRI and at mid-term vs. short-term MRI, paralleling results from large clinical trials. Conversely, no significant further benefit was evident at long-term radiological reassessment [14]. Persistent fistulous tracts were still detectable at MRI after a full year of therapy in nearly 80% of patients despite an almost equal percentage of patients with clinical benefit from infliximab. On the basis of these findings, Karmiris et al. questioned the possibility of complete fistula healing while acknowledging the value of MRI in treatment monitoring but only during the first year of treatment [14].

References

1. Hoeffel C, Arrive L, Mourra N, et al. (2006) Anatomic and pathologic findings at external phased-array pelvic MR imaging after surgery for anorectal disease. Radiographics 26:1391-1407
2. Tonolini M, Campari A, Bianco R (2011) Ileal pouch and related complications: spectrum of imaging findings with emphasis on MRI. Abdom Imaging 36:698-706
3. de Miguel Criado J, del Salto LG, Rivas PF, et al. (2012) MR imaging evaluation of perianal fistulas: spectrum of imaging features. Radiographics 32:175-194
4. Ng SC, Plamondon S, Gupta A, et al. (2009) Prospective evaluation of anti-tumor necrosis factor therapy guided by magnetic resonance imaging for Crohn's perineal fistulas. Am J Gastroenterol 104:2973-2986
5. Orlando A, Colombo E, Kohn A, et al. (2005) Infliximab in the treatment of Crohn's disease: predictors of response in an Italian multicentric open study. Dig Liver Dis 37:577-583
6. Bell SJ, Halligan S, Windsor AC, et al. (2003) Response of fistulating Crohn's disease to infliximab treatment assessed by magnetic resonance imaging. Aliment Pharmacol Ther 17:387-393
7. Schwartz DA (2009) Editorial: Imaging and the treatment of Crohn's perianal fistulas: to see is to believe. Am J Gastroenterol 104:2987-2989
8. Savoye-Collet C, Savoye G, Koning E, et al. (2010) Fistulizing perianal Crohn's disease: Contrast-enhanced magnetic resonance imaging assessment at 1 year on maintenance anti-TNF-alpha therapy. Inflamm Bowel Dis
9. Present DH, Rutgeerts P, Targan S, et al. (1999) Infliximab for the treatment of fistulas in patients with Crohn's disease. N Engl J Med 340:1398-1405
10. Van Assche G, Vanbeckevoort D, Bielen D, et al. (2003) Magnetic resonance imaging of the effects of infliximab on perianal fistulizing Crohn's disease. Am J Gastroenterol 98:332-339
11. Caprilli R, Gassull MA, Escher JC, et al. (2006) European evidence based consensus on the diagnosis and management of Crohn's disease: special situations. Gut 55 Suppl 1:i36-58
12. Osterman MT, Lichtenstein GR (2006) Infliximab in fistulizing Crohn's disease. Gastroenterol Clin North Am 35:795-820
13. Tougeron D, Savoye G, Savoye-Collet C, et al. (2009) Predicting factors of fistula healing and clinical remission after infliximab-based combined therapy for perianal fistulizing Crohn's disease. Dig Dis Sci 54:1746-1752
14. Karmiris K, Bielen D, Vanbeckevoort D, et al. (2011) Long-term monitoring of infliximab therapy for perianal fistulizing Crohn's disease by using magnetic resonance imaging. Clin Gastroenterol Hepatol 9:130-136

Ulcerative Colitis and Ileal Pouch Surgery

23

Massimo Tonolini

In the past, a greatly overestimated prevalence of perianal complications in patients with ulcerative colitis (UC), approaching 20–25%, was reported. Indeed, a large percentage of these patients had probably been misdiagnosed and were actually suffering from Crohn's disease or indeterminate colitis. Nonetheless, it is clear that perianal inflammatory disease sometimes occurs in the setting of UC [1].

The most common perianal conditions associated with UC include hemorrhoids and anal fissures, which are usually not assessed with imaging. Perianal and anovaginal fistulas, sometimes with abscess collections, have been reported in up to 5–6% of UC patients, are complex in nearly half the cases, and are strongly associated with distal or extensive active bowel disease [2]. Since perianal suppuration may remain undetected—with dangerous consequences—if symptoms are attributed to the primary intestinal disease, strong clinical awareness and prompt imaging assessment are needed to prevent local progression and distant sepsis. Furthermore, the same patients with severe UC are also at higher risk of anastomotic leakage and postoperative complications during proctocolectomy with ileal pouch–anal anastomosis (IPAA) surgery [1, 2]. In our experience, MRI performed with the same modality and protocol previously described for perianal Crohn's disease allows the confident detection and useful classification of perianal inflammatory disease also in patients with UC (Figs. 23.1, 23.2).

Currently, IPAA represents the surgical therapy of choice for refractory UC, preserving fecal continence and an acceptable lifestyle. After surgery, prolonged clinical and instrumental follow-up is recommended, considering the significant incidence of pouch-related complications: the long-term mor-

M. Tonolini (✉)
Radiology Department, Luigi Sacco University Hospital
Milan, Italy
e-mail: mtonolini@sirm.org

M.Tonolini and G. Maconi (eds.), *Imaging of Perianal Inflammatory Diseases*,
DOI: 10.1007/978-88-470-2847-0_23, © Springer-Verlag Italia 2013

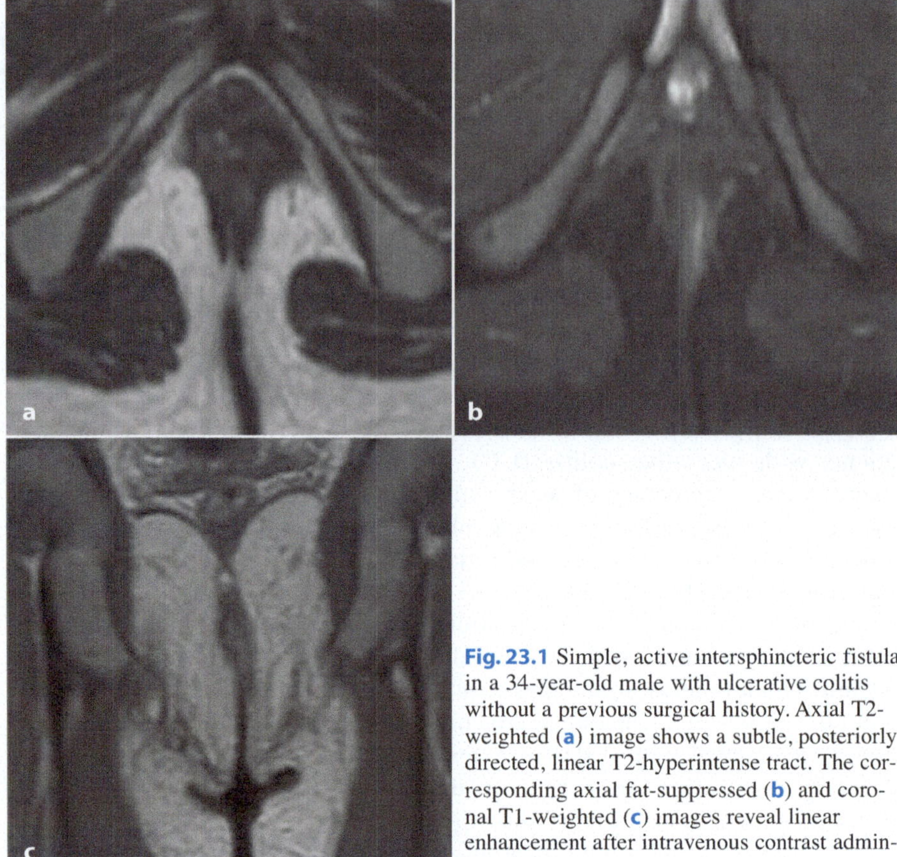

Fig. 23.1 Simple, active intersphincteric fistula in a 34-year-old male with ulcerative colitis without a previous surgical history. Axial T2-weighted (**a**) image shows a subtle, posteriorly directed, linear T2-hyperintense tract. The corresponding axial fat-suppressed (**b**) and coronal T1-weighted (**c**) images reveal linear enhancement after intravenous contrast administration

bidity approaches 70% after 10 years and a non-negligible rate of pouch failure can lead to pouch removal and permanent ileostomy [3-6].

A wide spectrum of pouch-related complications may be encountered, including pouchitis, anastomotic leakages and pelvic abscess collections, perianal or anovaginal fistulas, anal stenosis, and small bowel obstruction [3, 7-9]. Knowledge of surgical procedure details as well as the normal imaging appearance of the ileal pouch reservoir and the possible complications are required for confident interpretation of diagnostic studies in patients treated by IPAA [7].

Based on its wide availability and the very fast acquisition times of current multidetector scanners, CT is the mainstay imaging technique to assess clinically suspected complications during the early postoperative period in patients undergoing IPAA. Intravenous iodinated contrast medium is usually injected, whereas bowel opacification with water-soluble contrast per os or per rectum may prove useful for problem-solving or to rule out anastomotic leakage. At

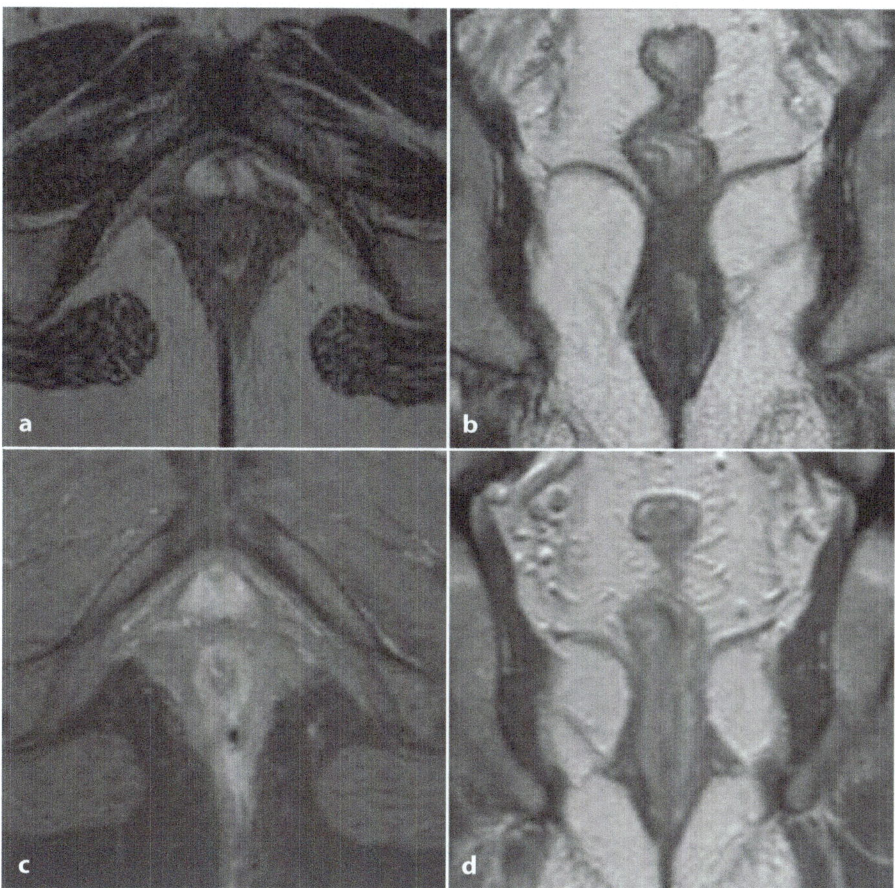

Fig. 23.2 A 40-year-old male with ulcerative colitis undergoing medical treatment. Axial (**a**) and coronal (**b**) T2-weighted images reveal an intersphincteric horseshoe-shaped collection. Axial fat-suppressed (**c**) and coronal (**d**) T1-weighted imaging after intravenous contrast result in active enhancement of the intersphincteric space and the posterior fistula. Clinical examination confirmed a draining orifice

CT, the ileal pouch reservoir is identified as a fluid-filled structure in the anatomical location of the resected rectum, with metallic surgical staples located 180° to each other. The pouch-anal anastomosis, indicated by the presence of hyperdense clips, should also be identified as its represents a possible source of leakage (Fig. 23.3). CT is reliable in the diagnosis of pouch-related septic complications, suggested by the detection of extraluminal air, fluid, or contrast material [9, 10].

More recently, pelvic MRI has been reported as a very accurate modality for the assessment of postoperative IPAA anatomy and possible complications. MRI is well tolerated even by patients with anal pain or stenosis, as the images

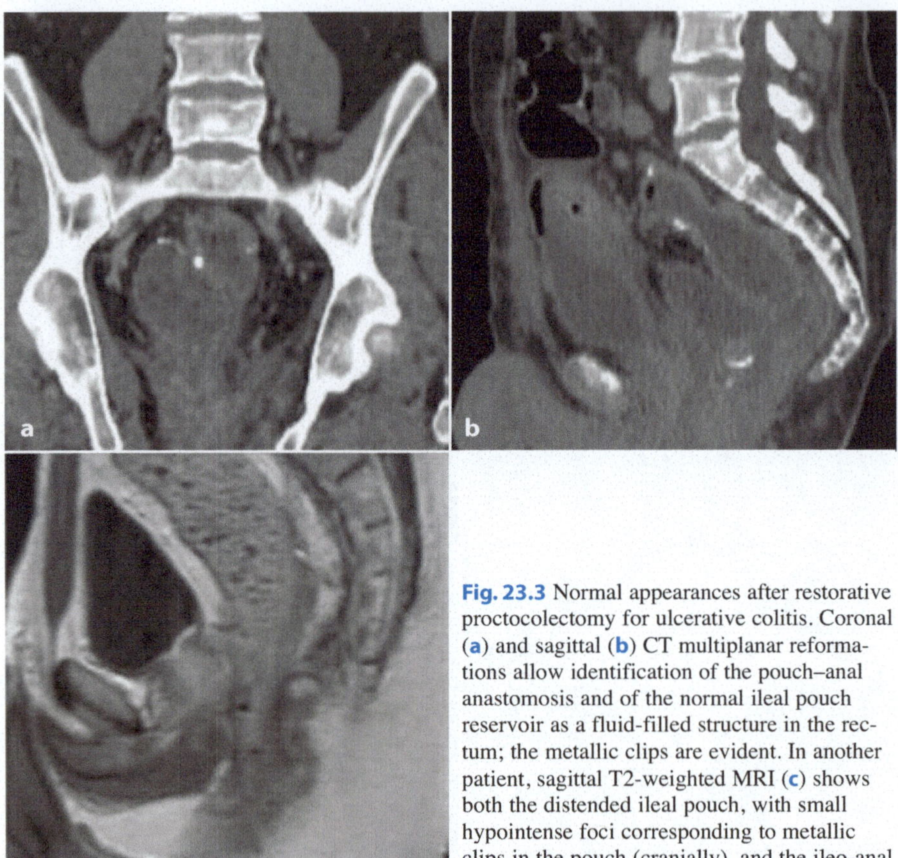

Fig. 23.3 Normal appearances after restorative proctocolectomy for ulcerative colitis. Coronal (**a**) and sagittal (**b**) CT multiplanar reformations allow identification of the pouch–anal anastomosis and of the normal ileal pouch reservoir as a fluid-filled structure in the rectum; the metallic clips are evident. In another patient, sagittal T2-weighted MRI (**c**) shows both the distended ileal pouch, with small hypointense foci corresponding to metallic clips in the pouch (cranially), and the ileo-anal anastomosis (caudally)

are acquired with external phased-array coils without special patient preparation. The lack of irradiation and limited biologic invasiveness of gadolinium contrast are particularly beneficial in young patients with chronic inflammatory bowel diseases, who often need imaging follow-up studies. Other significant advantages of MRI include panoramic and detailed views, a native multiplanar capability, and high contrast resolution [7-9].

At MRI, the normal ileal pouch reservoir is identified by the small hypointense ferromagnetic artifacts (signal voids) on all sequences, corresponding to the location of the metallic staples (Fig. 23.3). After IPAA surgery, UC patients may develop perianal fistulizing complications that are indistinguishable from those usually seen in Crohn's disease (Figs. 23.4, 23.5). Typically, active fistulous tracts appear as fluid-filled hyperintense tubular structures of variable length on high-resolution T2-weighted and STIR images. Abscess collections are easily identified, sometimes with air-fluid levels and mass

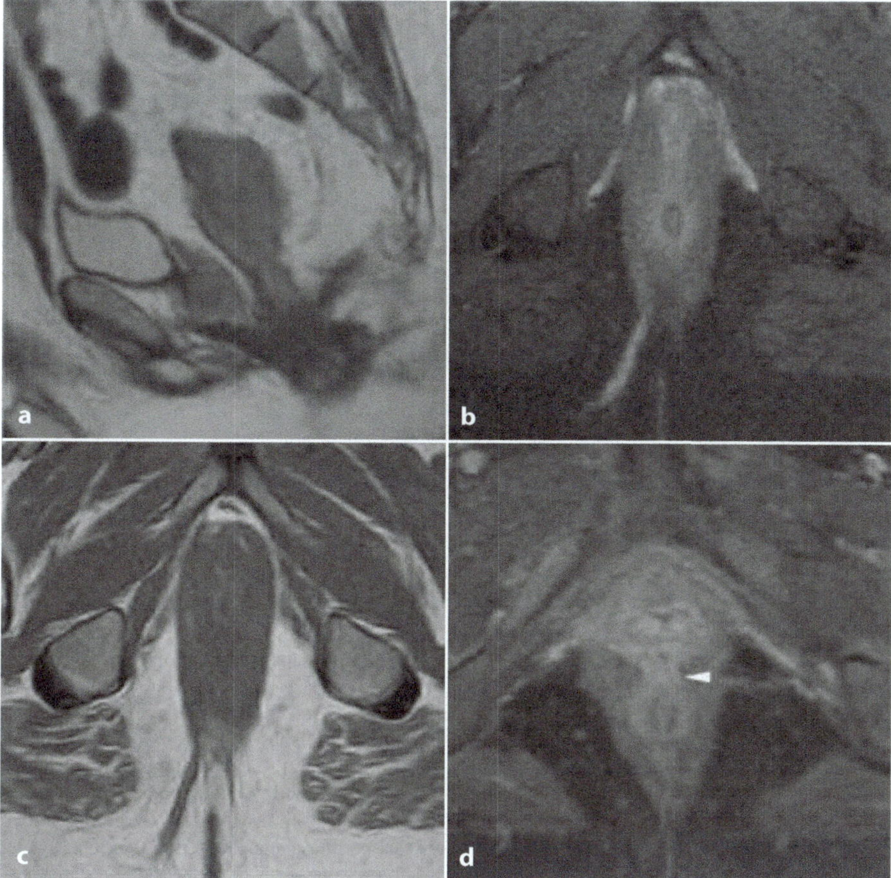

Fig. 23.4 A 47-year-old male patient with ulcerative colitis (UC) treated with IPAA. Sagittal (**a**) T2-weighted, axial STIR (**b**) and unenhanced T1-weighted (**c**) images allow identification of the ileal pouch and of a long, fluid-containing transsphincteric fistula crossing diagonally through the right ischioanal fossa. In another, female patient with UC, the axial contrast-enhanced fat-suppressed T1-weighted image (**d**) identifies an anovaginal fistula (*arrowhead*), clinically suspected due to a complaint of vaginal discharge

effect. Inflamed granulation tissue in the walls of abscesses and fistulas will positively enhance after intravenous gadolinium, whereas the contents of a purulent abscess and endoluminal fluid in fistulas remain T1-hypointense after contrast [7-9]. In such cases, a significant concern is usually raised regarding misinterpretation of the underlying disease as UC rather than Crohn's disease on the basis of clinical, endoscopic, imaging, and pathologic findings. In some series, including these comprising UC patients with perianal disease, reconsideration of histology specimens and examination of the small bowel generally excluded Crohn's disease whereas a modified diagnosis occurred in a few patients [2, 11, 12].

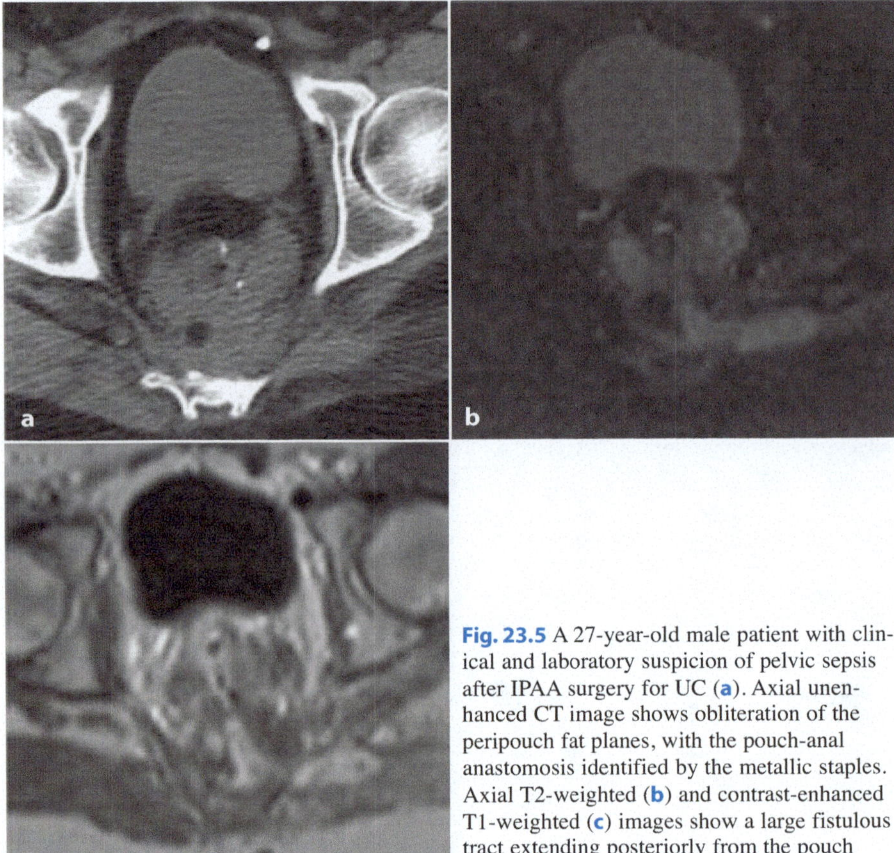

Fig. 23.5 A 27-year-old male patient with clinical and laboratory suspicion of pelvic sepsis after IPAA surgery for UC (**a**). Axial unenhanced CT image shows obliteration of the peripouch fat planes, with the pouch-anal anastomosis identified by the metallic staples. Axial T2-weighted (**b**) and contrast-enhanced T1-weighted (**c**) images show a large fistulous tract extending posteriorly from the pouch anastomosis towards the left gluteal region

Pouch-related pelvic sepsis has a variably reported incidence and a presentation similar to that of perianal inflammation, including local pain, purulent discharge, fever, and increased laboratory indicators of inflammation. Its identification is of paramount importance since it represents the most significant cause of pouch failure and reoperation in UC patients [3, 4]. Septic postoperative complications, most often related to pouch-anal anastomosis leakage, may give rise to fistulas and abscesses involving the peripouch and presacral fat planes, the ano-perianal region, urinary bladder, vagina, perineal skin, and subcutaneous tissues (Fig. 23.5) [7, 9]. In our experience, MRI has proved to be particularly valuable in the differentiation of pouch-related pelvic sepsis—even in patients with normal endoscopic findings—from simple pouchitis, which is the most common complication of IPAA surgery in UC patients [8]. The former usually requires an aggressive therapy whereas the latter is a nonspecific, idiopathic inflammation of the ileal reservoir that is successfully managed with medical therapy and associated with a good long-term prognosis, rarely leading to the need for surgical removal [5, 13, 14]. MRI features indicative of uncomplicated pouchitis include pouch wall thickening (> 2 mm) and enhancement, usually associated with lymphadenopathies (at least 3 peripouch nodes or one > 1 cm) and variable proliferation and stranding of the peripouch fat [7, 15].

References

1. Hamzaoglu I, Hodin RA (2005) Perianal problems in patients with ulcerative colitis. Inflamm Bowel Dis 11:856-859
2. Zabana Y, Van Domselaar M, Garcia-Planella E, et al (2011) Perianal disease in patients with ulcerative colitis: A case-control study. J Crohns Colitis 5:338-341
3. Beliard A, Prudhomme M (2010) Ileal reservoir with ileo-anal anastomosis: long-term complications. J Visc Surg 147:e137-144
4. Fazio VW, Ziv Y, Church JM, et al (1995) Ileal pouch-anal anastomoses complications and function in 1005 patients. Ann Surg 222:120-127
5. Hahnloser D, Pemberton JH, Wolff BG, et al (2007) Results at up to 20 years after ileal pouch-anal anastomosis for chronic ulcerative colitis. Br J Surg 94:333-340
6. Hueting WE, Buskens E, van der Tweel I, et al (2005) Results and complications after ileal pouch anal anastomosis: a meta-analysis of 43 observational studies comprising 9,317 patients. Dig Surg 22:69-79
7. Broder JC, Tkacz JN, Anderson SW, et al (2010) Ileal pouch-anal anastomosis surgery: imaging and intervention for post-operative complications. Radiographics 30:221-233
8. Tonolini M, Campari A, Bianco R (2011) Ileal pouch and related complications: spectrum of imaging findings with emphasis on MRI. Abdom Imaging 36:698-706
9. Crema MD, Richarme D, Azizi L, et al (2006) Pouchography, CT, and MRI features of ileal J pouch-anal anastomosis. AJR Am J Roentgenol 187:W594-603
10. Seggerman RE, Chen MY, Waters GS, et al (2003) Pictorial essay. Radiology of ileal pouch-anal anastomosis surgery. AJR Am J Roentgenol 180:999-1002
11. Viscido A, Habib FI, Kohn A, et al (2003) Infliximab in refractory pouchitis complicated by fistulae following ileo-anal pouch for ulcerative colitis. Aliment Pharmacol Ther 17:1263-1271
12. Goldstein NS, Sanford WW, Bodzin JH (1997) Crohn's-like complications in patients with ulcerative colitis after total proctocolectomy and ileal pouch-anal anastomosis. Am J Surg Pathol 21:1343-1353
13. Cheifetz A, Itzkowitz S (2004) The diagnosis and treatment of pouchitis in inflammatory bowel disease. J Clin Gastroenterol 38:S44-50
14. Simchuk EJ, Thirlby RC (2000) Risk factors and true incidence of pouchitis in patients after ileal pouch-anal anastomoses. World J Surg 24:851-856
15. Nadgir RN, Soto JA, Dendrinos K, et al (2006) MRI of complicated pouchitis. AJR Am J Roentgenol 187:W386-391

Cryptogenic Fistulas

24

Massimo Tonolini

In the surgical literature, cryptoglandular fistulas and abscesses are invariably separated from perianal Crohn's disease based on fundamental differences in their respective epidemiology, etiology, pathology, and surgical treatment. Conversely, in most radiological publications, the same distinction is usually absent, since the imaging appearances of these entities are usually considered similar or indistinguishable [1].

As extensively discussed in previous chapters of this book, perianal inflammation occurs in nearly half of Crohn's disease patients, as a result of chronic granulomatous transmural inflammation. In the general population, fistula-in-ano is a relatively uncommon condition, with an estimated incidence of 1:10,000 individuals, most often affecting adult males [2, 3]. Unlike Crohn's perianal disease, nonspecific cryptogenic fistulas arise as a consequence of localized infection originating in the anal crypts and glands located at the level of the dentate line, possibly promoted by events such as acute diarrhea or trauma. When purulent debris obstructs the draining duct, gland infection gives rise to an intersphincteric abscess, which if left untreated may lead to the development of a fistula [1, 4].

The pathologic features of cryptoglandular inflammation that are distinct from those of perianal Crohn's disease are particularly relevant for diagnostic imaging. Briefly, perianal fistulas may be described as channels of variable diameter lined by epithelium and granulation tissue, crossing from an internal orifice in the anus to an external one on the cutaneous surface. At surgical examination, the inner opening of a cryptogenic fistula is invariably along the dentate line, in the intermediate portion of the anal canal at the transition between columnar and squamous epithelium, most commonly in the 6 o'clock

M. Tonolini (✉)
Radiology Department, Luigi Sacco University Hospital
Milan, Italy
e-mail: mtonolini@sirm.org

M.Tonolini and G. Maconi (eds.), *Imaging of Perianal Inflammatory Diseases*,
DOI: 10.1007/978-88-470-2847-0_24, © Springer-Verlag Italia 2013

position given that anal glands are more numerous posteriorly [4]. The typical cryptoglandular fistula consists of a small primary tract located close to the anal sphincter complex and an external opening; complex features such as secondary tracts, horseshoe spread, and abscess collections are rarely present [1]. At histological comparison, significant differences in the cellular composition of cryptoglandular and Crohn's fistulas have been reported: in the former, granulation tissue densely populated by macrophages surrounds the epithelium, whereas in the latter T- and B-lymphocyte infiltration predominates [5].

As previously discussed for Crohn's perianal inflammatory disease, MRI is currently the imaging modality of choice to assess the topography of clinically diagnosed fistulous tracts and the possible presence of abscess collections, with excellent diagnostic results related to the high spatial and contrast resolution, panoramic view, and multiplanar capabilities [4, 6, 7].

At MRI, cryptoglandular fistulas are visualized as tubular structures of variable length and diameter, rarely multiple or branching, with an internal canal of

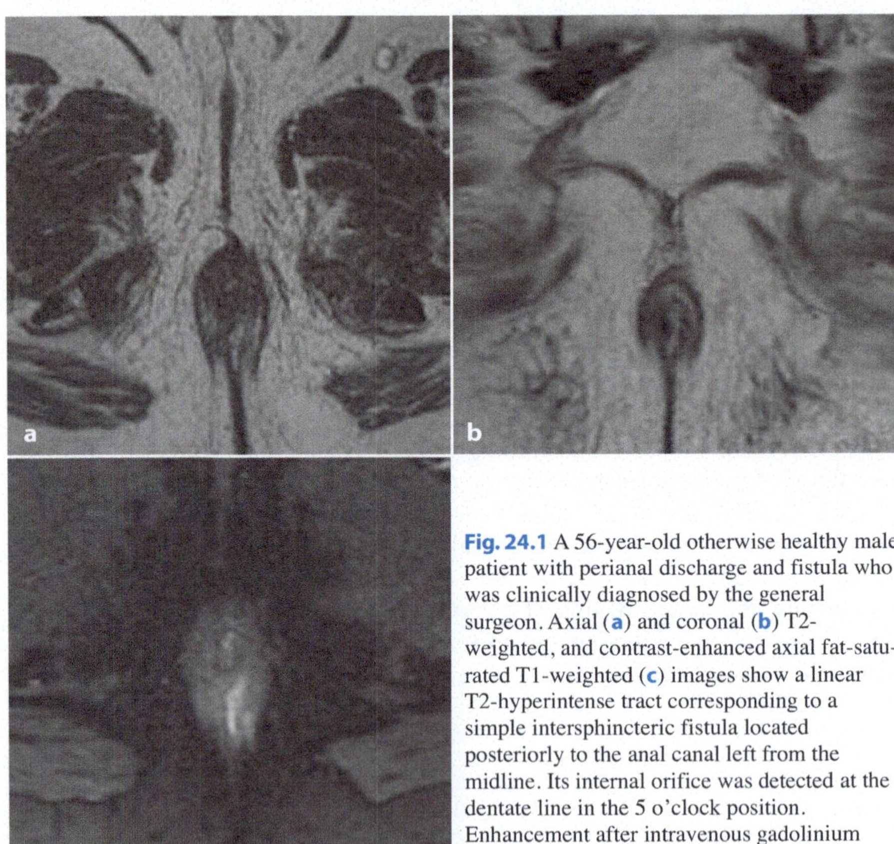

Fig. 24.1 A 56-year-old otherwise healthy male patient with perianal discharge and fistula who was clinically diagnosed by the general surgeon. Axial (**a**) and coronal (**b**) T2-weighted, and contrast-enhanced axial fat-saturated T1-weighted (**c**) images show a linear T2-hyperintense tract corresponding to a simple intersphincteric fistula located posteriorly to the anal canal left from the midline. Its internal orifice was detected at the dentate line in the 5 o'clock position. Enhancement after intravenous gadolinium along the fistulous tract is consistent with active inflammation

hyperintense signal as seen on high-resolution T2-weighted images. This area of hyperintensity corresponds to the true lumen and granulation tissue. There may also be a peripheral wall of relatively lower signal intensity and consisting of partly fibrotic tissue (Fig. 24.1). On T1-weighted sequences, transsphincteric fistulas are identified as hypointense tracts crossing the ischioanal fatty space.

Imaging signs that are generally consistent with inflammatory activity include fluid-like hyperintensity on T2-weighted images and the enhancement of granulation tissue in fistulous walls observed on post-gadolinium contrast T1-weighted sequences (Fig. 24.1). Similarly, abscesses are identified as strongly hyperintense collections on T2 and STIR sequences due to their purulent and debris content, with strong enhancement along the periphery best visualized on fat-suppressed T1-weighted images acquired after intravenous contrast. When present, the unusual gas content is better visualized on CT scans than by MRI (Fig. 24.2). Chronic, inactive fistulas show low signal intensity on T2-weighted and STIR images due to the progressive development of fibrosis [1-3, 7].

In our experience, cryptogenic fistulas, which are most often simple and predominantly located in close proximity to the anal canal, can be conveniently staged following the same classifications proposed for perianal Crohn's disease, namely, the anatomic scheme of Parks (developed according to surgical findings) and the MRI-based system of St James' University Hospital [1, 3, 8, 9].

After the initial report by Lunniss et al., in which MRI was shown to be the most accurate method for determining the presence and course of anal fistulas, other authors confirmed the relative inaccuracy of surgical exploration and, instead, the ability of MRI to identify clinically undetected perianal inflammation, thus leading to an altered surgical management of these patients and a reduction of postoperative recurrences [10-12]. Currently, there is overwhelming evidence that the additional value of MRI compared to clinical assessment allows correct surgical planning and improves the clinical outcome [4]. In patients with Crohn's perianal inflammatory disease, this conclusion has been confirmed by a statistically significant difference, given that Crohn's-related fistulas tend to be complex, with secondary tracts and multiple abscesses, and are therefore not easily assessed clinically. In these patients, an inaccurate preoperative evaluation often leads to treatment failure, since unrecognized lesions are more likely to be incompletely treated and thus to subsequently recur [1].

A similar benefit from preoperative MRI is not consistently obtained with cryptogenic fistulas since the majority of them are simple, without branching secondary tracts or abscesses [1, 3, 13]. In patients who do not have Crohn's disease, MRI is therefore recommended to assess recurrent perianal inflammatory disease and clinical suspicion of complex fistulization and/or abscess [3]. MRI can prove useful in the comprehensive preoperative visualization of disease extent when uncertainty exists about the optimal surgical approach, e.g., fistulotomy vs. seton placement. Furthermore, due to its reproducibility, MRI can confidently re-assess perianal inflammatory disease after medical treatment and surgical procedures [1, 4].

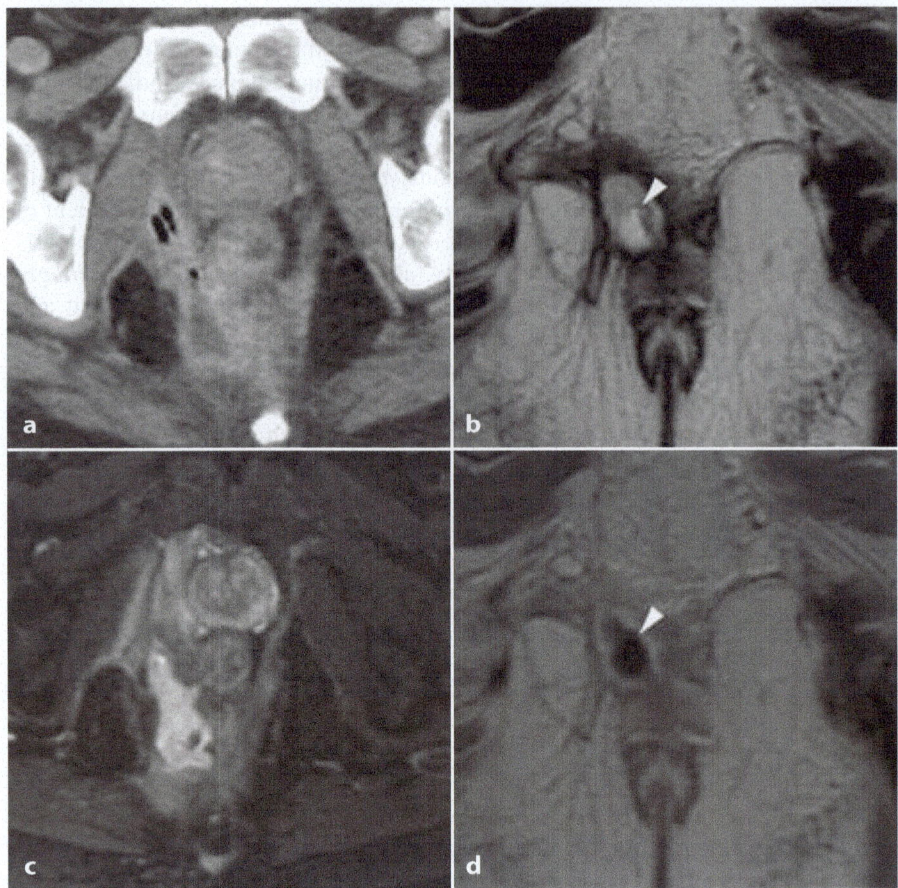

Fig. 24.2 A 73-year-old male hospitalized patient who underwent CT for abdominal disease complaints unrelated to the anorectal tract. Axial contrast-enhanced CT image (**a**) detects a sizeable abscess collection with peripheral enhancement, mixed air, and fluid content occupying the right ischioanal space. MRI was requested to stage the perianal inflammatory disease: coronal T2-weighted (**b**), axial STIR (**c**), and contrast-enhanced coronal T1-weighted (**d**) images show an abscess collection involving the right levator ani muscle, originating from an ipsilateral fistulous tract and drained by means of a positioned Foley catheter (balloon indicated by arrowheads). A blind-ending secondary tract crosses downwards in the ipsilateral ischioanal space

References

1. Hussain SM, Outwater EK, Joekes EC, et al (2000) Clinical and MR imaging features of cryptoglandular and Crohn's fistulas and abscesses. Abdom Imaging 25:67-74
2. Torkzad MR, U. K (2011) MRI for assessment of anal fistula. Insights Imaging 1:62-71
3. Ziech M, Felt-Bersma R, Stoker J (2009) Imaging of perianal fistulas. Clin Gastroenterol Hepatol 7:1037-1045
4. Halligan S, Stoker J (2006) Imaging of fistula in ano. Radiology 239:18-33

5. Bataille F, Klebl F, Rummele P, et al (2004) Morphological characterisation of Crohn's disease fistulae. Gut 53:1314-1321
6. Maccioni F, Colaiacomo MC, Stasolla A, et al (2002) Value of MRI performed with phased-array coil in the diagnosis and pre-operative classification of perianal and anal fistulas. Radiol Med 104:58-67
7. Szurowska E, Wypych J, Izycka-Swieszewska E (2007) Perianal fistulas in Crohn's disease: MRI diagnosis and surgical planning : MRI in fistulizing perianal Crohn's disease. Abdom Imaging 32:705-718
8. Parks AG (1961) Pathogenesis and treatment of fistula-in-ano. Br Med J 1:463-469
9. Morris J, Spencer JA, Ambrose NS (2000) MR imaging classification of perianal fistulas and its implications for patient management. Radiographics 20:623-635; discussion 635-627
10. Lunniss PJ, Faris B, Rees HC, et al (1993) Histological and microbiological assessment of the role of microorganisms in chronic anal fistula. Br J Surg 80:1072
11. Buchanan G, Halligan S, Williams A, et al (2002) Effect of MRI on clinical outcome of recurrent fistula-in-ano. Lancet 360:1661-1662
12. Spencer JA, Ward J, Beckingham IJ, et al (1996) Dynamic contrast-enhanced MR imaging of perianal fistulas. AJR Am J Roentgenol 167:735-741
13. Beets-Tan RG, Beets GL, van der Hoop AG, et al (2001) Preoperative MR imaging of anal fistulas: Does it really help the surgeon? Radiology 218:75-84

Sexually Transmitted Diseases 25

Massimo Tonolini

During the last few decades, there has been a steady increase in the incidence of sexually transmitted diseases, attributed to risky sexual behaviors. From a practical point of view, sexually transmitted infections should always be suspected in patients with symptoms or abnormalities involving the anorectal region and who have a positive history of anal intercourse [1].

Individuals infected with the human immunodeficiency virus (HIV) are particularly prone to develop pathologic conditions of the anorectal tract, which are reported to occur in approximately a third of this population [2, 3]. Perianal diseases are by far the most prevalent (75–90% of cases) in HIV-positive male homosexuals, who often have a history of other sexually transmitted diseases (45% of patients). Symptoms involving the perineal region (such as local pain or pruritus, constipation, mass, purulent secretions, rectal or fecal bleeding) may significantly compromise the quality of life of these patients [3].

Perianal disease in patients with acquired immunodeficiency syndrome (AIDS) is often complex and varied, including multiple associated conditions that are difficult to treat, have prolonged healing times, and commonly recur. Clinical and/or surgical attention may be sought throughout the course of the systemic disease. In 5% of cases, early perianal manifestations may lead to the initial suspicion or diagnosis of HIV infection [3].

In HIV patients, a wide spectrum of related perianal conditions may be found. Conventional, benign non-infectious disorders, including anal fissures, ulcers, and hemorrhoids, are diagnosed in 64% of patients. None of these disorders are usually investigated with imaging modalities.

Fistulas and abscesses occur frequently in individuals who practice receptive anal intercourse. Bacteria isolated from the infected sites include

M. Tonolini (✉)
Radiology Department, Luigi Sacco University Hospital
Milan, Italy
e-mail: mtonolini@sirm.org

M.Tonolini and G. Maconi (eds.), *Imaging of Perianal Inflammatory Diseases*,
DOI: 10.1007/978-88-470-2847-0_25, © Springer-Verlag Italia 2013

Escherichia coli, *Klebsiella*, and *Enterococcus*. In this setting, cross-sectional imaging with CT or MRI may be requested to assess the topography and extent of perianal infections, particularly to confirm or exclude the presence of purulent collections (Figs. 25.1, 25.2) in order to allow correct surgical planning, since untreated perianal sepsis may sometimes lead to severe life-threatening complications such as disseminated sepsis or necrotizing fasciitis [3]. MRI better depicts the inflammatory changes and abscess collections and demonstrates their anatomical relationship to the sphincter complex, whereas CT acquisition is mostly employed in the urgent setting and may be usefully complemented with multiplanar reformations, which yield MRI-like anatomical information.

Venereal diseases (occurring in 56% of patients) include condylomas, syphilis (Fig. 25.2), gonorrhea, *Chlamydia*, and amebiasis, along with other peculiar HIV-associated infections such as cytomegalovirus (CMV), herpes simplex virus (HSV), and candidiasis [2, 3]. Globally, the most frequent diseases are condylomas (usually associated with oral and/or genital lesions) and ulcers (related to HSV and CMV infections) [2]. In Western countries, an increase in syphilis, mostly due to homosexual contacts, was recently reported. The variable and unspecific symptoms of syphilis consist of local pain sometimes associated with itching, tenesmus, urgency of defecation, or anal discharge, which may be purulent, mucoid, or blood-stained. Therefore, this uncommon diagnosis should be suspected in a patient who presents with anorectal lesions and particularly in active homosexual males [1, 4, 5].

Opportunistic intestinal infections account for a large proportion of the morbidity in HIV-infected patients and are usually assessed by means of microbiological and parasitic stool cultures coupled with endoscopy [9].

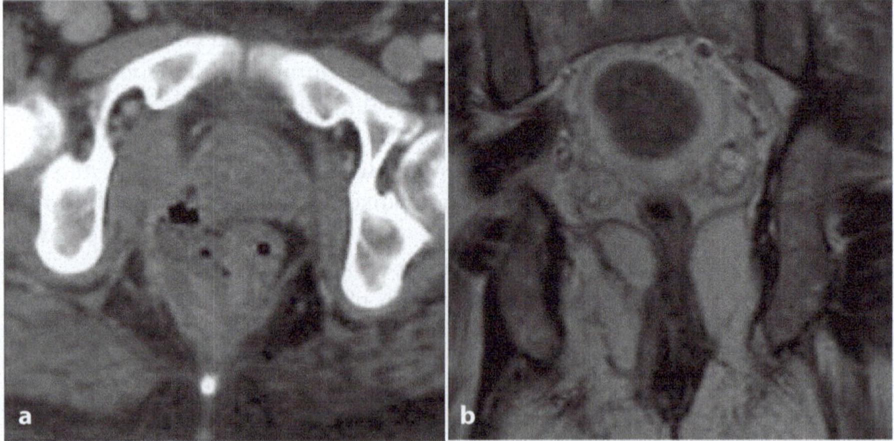

Fig. 25.1 A 40-year-old male HIV-infected patient hospitalized with sepsis. The caudalmost image from a total body CT (**a**) shows a right perianal abscess collection with fluid content and gas bubbles. Focused MRI better confirms the abscess process, which involves the right ischioanal fossa and levator ani muscle, as seen on the coronal T2-weighted image (**b**)

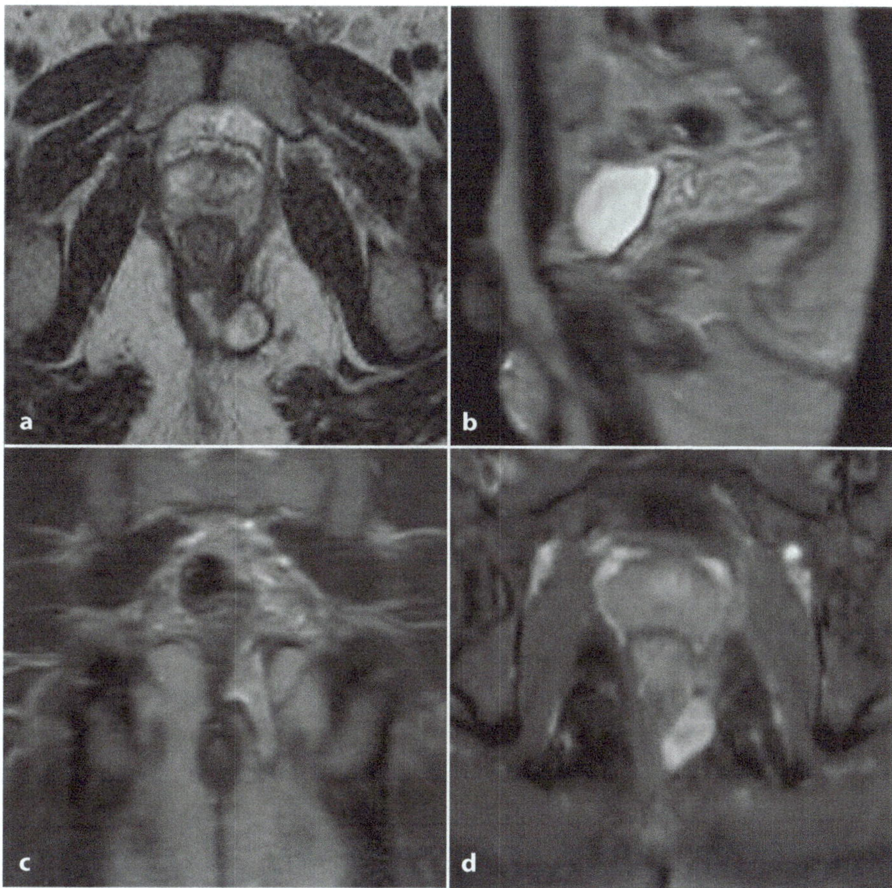

Fig. 25.2 A 37-year-old HIV-infected male homosexual with a clinical diagnosis of anal condylomas. Axial (**a**), sagittal (**b**), and coronal (**c**) T2-weighted images show a posterior perianal fistula and an abscess collection with involvement of the levator ani muscle; there is a secondary tract in the ischioanal space. On contrast-enhanced axial fat-suppressed (**d**) T1-weighted MRI, the left perianal abscess markedly enhances. Biopsy disclosed coexistent syphilis infection

Diagnostic imaging procedures, particularly MRI, may have a role in visualizing abnormalities involving the anorectal tract, inflammatory lesions and their topography, and possible complications such as abscess collections, as well as in differentiating benign lesions from solid neoplastic ones [10].

Although uncommon (about 7% of cases), anal tumors are more prevalent in HIV-infected patients than in the general population. They mainly consist of squamous-cell carcinomas associated with HPV infection, Kaposi's sarcoma, and, rarely, non-Hodgkin lymphoma [2, 3]. On CT, neoplastic lesions appear as solid soft-tissue thickenings or masses; on MRI, they are solid, T1-hypointense lesions with positive contrast enhancement, and of intermediate-to high signal intensity (usually heterogeneous in larger lesions) on T2-weighted and STIR images. In the imaging of HIV-infected patients, special attention should be paid to the presence of solid, enhancing tissue consistent with tumor as this finding indicates the need for biopsy (Fig. 25.3). Furthermore, as described elsewhere in this book, MRI allows convenient staging and post-treatment reassessment of anal neoplasms (Fig. 25.4).

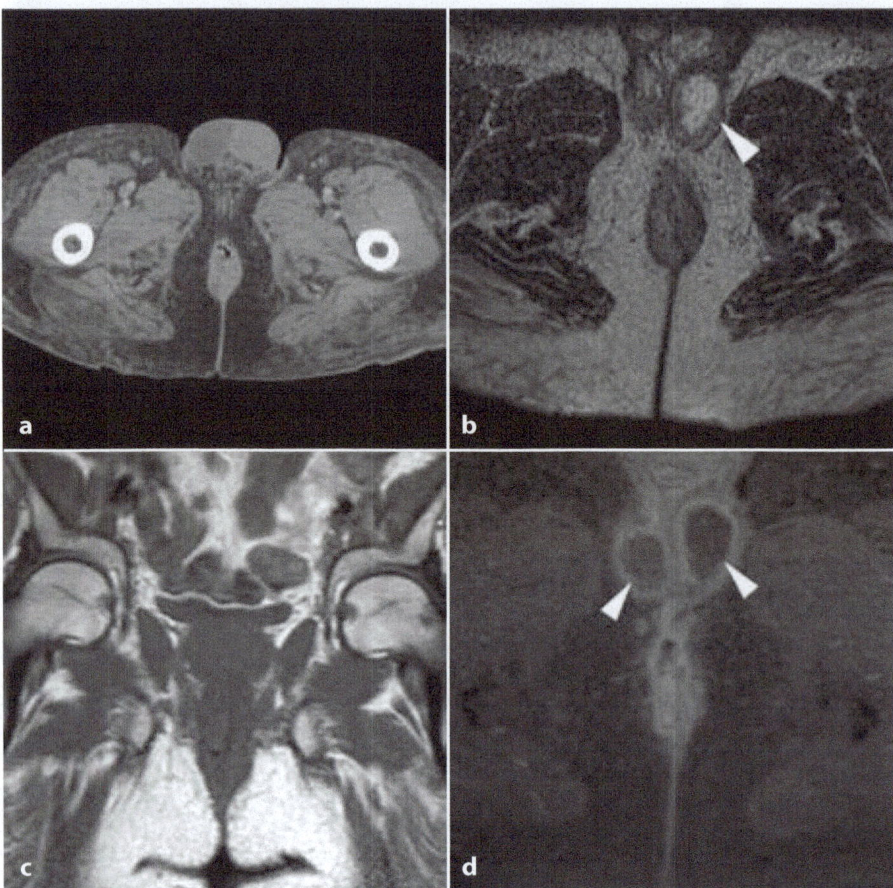

Fig. 25.3 A 41-year-old HIV-infected transsexual male hospitalized with sepsis. The caudalmost image from a body CT (**a**) shows a circumferential mural thickening of the anus. Focused MRI, including axial T2-weighted (**b**), unenhanced coronal (**c**), and contrast-enhanced fat-suppressed axial (**d**) images, confirm mural thickening of the anal canal, with hyperintense solid tissue more pronounced on the left side and probable ventral fistulization giving rise to the subcutaneous rim-enhancing abscess collection (*arrowheads*). Biopsy confirmed anal carcinoma

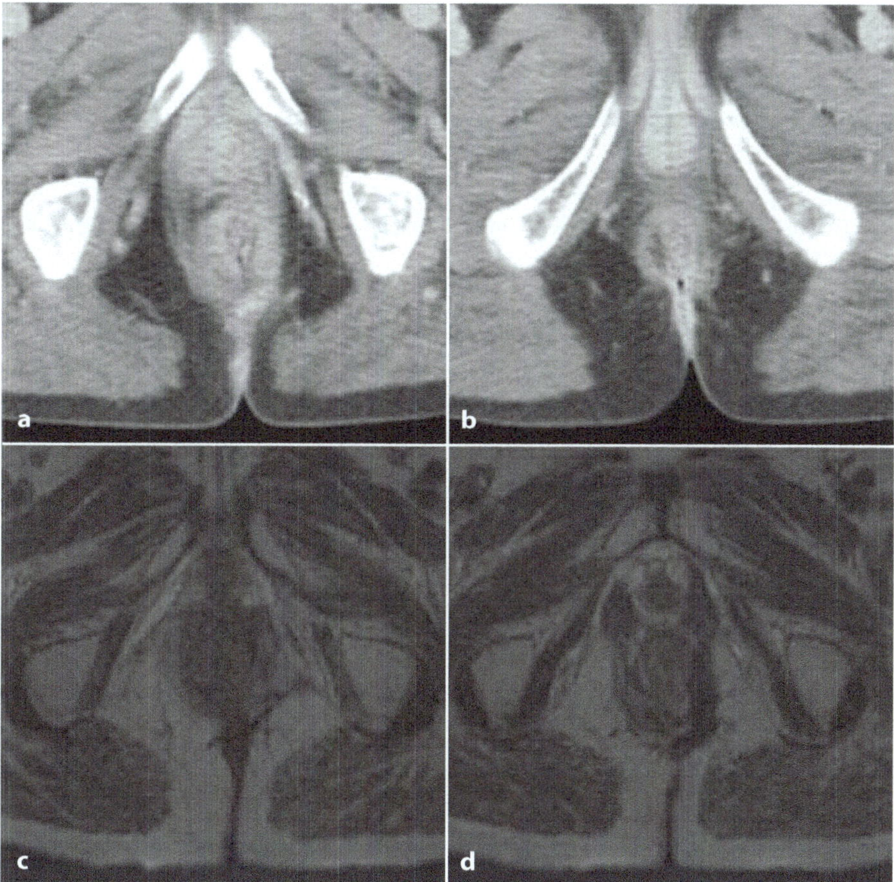

Fig. 25.4 A 58-year-old male with long-standing AIDS. The caudalmost images from a body CT (**a**, **b**) unexpectedly revealed left-sided solid mural thickening of the anus, associated with a posterior fistula. Axial T2-weighted images from initial (**a**) and follow-up (**b**) MRI studies, respectively, detect invasion of the ipsilateral ischioanal fossa by hyperintense tissue, corresponding to biopsy-proven squamous-cell carcinoma, and the appearance of low-signal intensity fibrosis following chemoradiotherapy, with a probable persistent neoplastic nodule dorsally

References

1. Wexner SD (1990) Sexually transmitted diseases of the colon, rectum, and anus. The challenge of the nineties. Dis Colon Rectum 33:1048-1062
2. Nadal SR, Manzione CR, Galvao VM, et al (1999) Perianal diseases in HIV-positive patients compared with a seronegative population. Dis Colon Rectum 42:649-654
3. Barrett WL, Callahan TD, Orkin BA (1998) Perianal manifestations of human immunodeficiency virus infection: experience with 260 patients. Dis Colon Rectum 41:606-611; discussion 611-602

4. Cha JM, Choi SI, Lee JI (2010) Rectal syphilis mimicking rectal cancer. Yonsei Med J 51:276-278
5. Song SH, Jang I, Kim BS, et al (2005) A case of primary syphilis in the rectum. J Korean Med Sci 20:886-887
6. Pritt BS, Clark CG (2008) Amebiasis. Mayo Clin Proc 83:1154-1159; quiz 1159-1160
7. Park MS, Kim KW, Ha HK, et al (2008) Intestinal parasitic infection. Abdom Imaging 33:166-171
8. Alavi KA (2007) Amebiasis. Clin Colon Rectal Surg 20:33-37
9. Kuhlman JE, Fishman EK (1990) Acute abdomen in AIDS: CT diagnosis and triage. Radiographics 10:621-634
10. Hoeffel CC, Azizi L, Mourra N, et al (2006) MRI of rectal disorders. AJR Am J Roentgenol 187:W275-284
11. Yilmaz M, Memisoglu R, Aydin S, et al (2011) Anorectal syphilis mimicking Crohn's disease. J Infect Chemother
12. Hardin RE, Ferzli GS, Zenilman ME, et al (2007) Invasive amebiasis and ameboma formation presenting as a rectal mass: An uncommon case of malignant masquerade at a western medical center. World J Gastroenterol 13:5659-5661
13. Gulek B, Onel S (1999) US and CT findings of rectal amebian abscess. Eur Radiol 9:719-720

Cancer in Perianal Fistulas

26

Massimo Tonolini

Cancer of the anal canal is most often diagnosed in the sixth and seventh decades of life, with a pronounced female predominance. It is an uncommon disease that accounts for less than 2% of all gastrointestinal malignancies and only 5% of anorectal tumors, but according to recent reports its incidence is increasing [1-3]. Predisposing factors include previous pelvic therapeutic irradiation, Crohn's disease, and human immunodeficiency virus (HIV) infection. There is also a strong association between anal cancer, human papillomavirus (HPV) infection (detected in up to 70% of patients), and cervical cancer [2].

Carcinoma of the lower rectum and anus may complicate perianal Crohn's disease in up to 0.7% of patients. A higher risk is related to an early onset and a prolonged duration (15 years on average) of chronic inflammatory bowel disease. Conversely, the development of carcinoma in an anorectal fistula is exceptional in the absence of Crohn's disease [4]. The causal relationship between anorectal fistulas and cancer remains unclear. Neoplastic changes may occur secondary to constant mucosal regeneration; alternatively, fistulas may provide HPV with an easier access to the epithelial layers [4, 5]. Complex inflammation, with stricture and local pain, can hamper the clinical diagnosis of cancer arising in a patient with perianal Crohn's disease. Indeed, in most patients in the largest reported series the diagnosis was either delayed or unsuspected. Therefore, in Crohn's patients with early-onset or long-standing disease, a modification in symptoms or the appearance of new complaints should be investigated with care, including imaging and biopsy as needed, to avoid the misdiagnosis of cancer [4-6].

Histologically, the vast majority of anal tumors are squamous cell carcinomas, with adenocarcinomas constituting the remaining 10% [1]. Anal cancer is

M. Tonolini (✉)
Radiology Department, Luigi Sacco University Hospital
Milan, Italy
e-mail: mtonolini@sirm.org

M.Tonolini and G. Maconi (eds.), *Imaging of Perianal Inflammatory Diseases*,
DOI: 10.1007/978-88-470-2847-0_26,

an indolent, locally extensive disease with a propensity for lymphatic spread in a pattern depending on the location of the primary lesion within the anal canal. Lymphatic drainage from lesions distal to the dentate line is directed to the inguinal lymph nodes; conversely, the perirectal, internal iliac, and retroperitoneal lymph nodes are involved when the primary tumor arises above the dentate line [3, 7].

Due to its favorable anatomic location, anal cancer is usually detected clinically whereas imaging is needed to evaluate the local extent of the lesion, lymph node involvement, and the possible invasion of adjacent organs [1]. In patients undergoing imaging evaluation for perianal Crohn's inflammatory disease, the detection of solid tissue on CT or MRI scans should be reported as suspicious for neoplasm and a biopsy consequently suggested (Fig. 26.1).

In the presence of lesions of the anal canal, imaging techniques that include endoanal sonography and MRI probes are hampered by the pain experienced by the patient and by technical difficulties during probe positioning. Furthermore, endoanal imaging combines a very high degree of spatial detail with a limited field-of-view that does not allow comprehensive assessment of lymphatic spread [7]. Although CT may visualize anal cancers, MRI performed using external phased-array coils is the imaging modality of choice to assess primary treated lesions as well as recurrent ones, thus allowing pretreatment staging and radiotherapy planning [1, 7]. The acquisition protocols are mostly similar to those described for perianal inflammatory disease and rely heavily on multiplanar T2 sequences. The only important difference consists

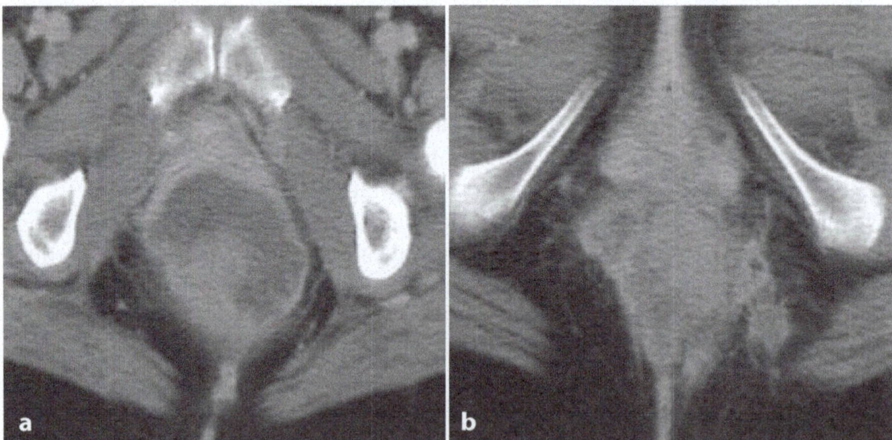

Fig. 26.1 A 38-year-old female patient with long-standing Crohn's disease, and previous surgical treatment for anovaginal fistula and abscess was investigated due to anal swelling and bleeding. Clinical examination disclosed perianal fistulous tracts with purulent secretion. Contrast-enhanced CT images (**a**, **b**) show an inhomogeneous, largely necrotic mass centered in the anus, associated with fluid-containing fistulous tracts in the left ischioanal space. Mucinous adenocarcinoma was treated with abdominoperineal anorectal amputation

of the usual lack of post-gadolinium sequences since according to most centers contrast-enhanced MRI acquisitions do not add significant information to those obtained from the intrinsic tissue contrast of high-resolution T2-weighted images [2, 7].

MRI provides a detailed visualization of the anal canal and nearby anatomic structures, with the notable exception that the dentate line is not recognizable. Neoplastic processes show low or intermediate T1 signal intensity and

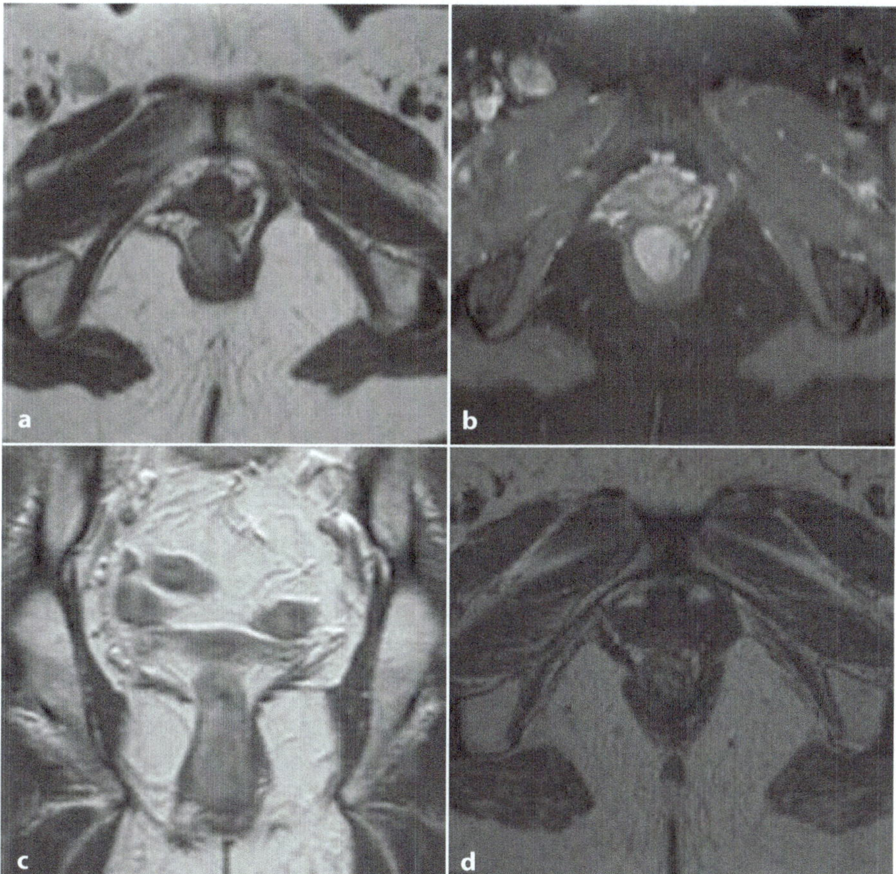

Fig. 26.2 A 46-year-old female patient with clinical and biopsy diagnosis of squamous cell anal carcinoma. MRI was requested to stage the disease. Axial T2-weighted (**a**), contrast-enhanced axial fat-saturated (**b**), and coronal (**c**) T1-weighted images after intravenous gadolinium show eccentric mural thickening of the anus with increased T2 signal intensity and strong homogeneous contrast enhancement with a maximum longitudinal diameter measuring 3 cm. Right inguinal adenopathy, with analogous signal and enhancement features consistent with nodal metastasis was determined. Following chemoradiotherapy, the axial T2-weighted image (**d**) shows the near-complete disappearance of both the anal neoplastic solid tissue and the lymphadenopathy

positive, usually intense enhancement after intravenous gadolinium contrast [1, 7]. On T2-weighted and STIR sequences, tumor tissue has an intermediate signal intensity, lower than that of normal ischioanal fat and almost always higher than the internal reference standard, i.e., uninvolved anal sphincters and gluteal muscles (Fig. 26.2) [1, 2].

In 2010, the European Society for Medical Oncology (ESMO) recommended MRI as the primary imaging modality for staging anal carcinoma [8]. Accurate staging is essential in terms of providing prognostic information and in guiding the correct therapeutic choice. It is based on the UICC/AJCC TNM classification shown in Table 26.1. Parameters to be assessed by imaging include the size of the primary lesion, the presence of metastasis in the perirectal, inguinal, or internal iliac lymph nodes, and possible invasion of the adjacent organs. At initial presentation half of the patients have shown a superficial (up to T2) tumor and 25% of them regional lymph node involvement [2, 7].

The sensitivity of MRI in the detection of anal cancer reportedly approaches 100% vs. 88.9% with endoscopic ultrasound (EUS). The latter is more accurate for smaller, superficial tumors; the same study reported that the two modalities may be considered complementary since EUS allows accurate T parameter staging, whereas MRI is needed to assess regional lymphadenopathies [9]. Since size criteria are inaccurate, the specificity for nodal evaluation can be improved by carefully observing the signal intensity features of lymph nodes: metastatic nodes usually have T1 and T2 signal intensities analogous to those of the primary tumor (Fig. 26.2) [7].

Table 26.1 TNM staging of anal cancer

Primary tumor (T)	
TX	Primary tumor cannot be assessed
T0	No evidence of primary tumor
T1	Tumor ≤ 2 cm in its greatest dimension
T2	Tumor 2–5 cm in its greatest dimension
T3	Tumor > 5 cm in its greatest dimension
T4	Tumor of any size invading adjacent organ(s), e.g., vagina, urethra, bladder
Regional lymph nodes (N)	
NX	Regional lymph nodes cannot be assessed
N0	No regional lymph node metastasis
N1	Metastasis in perirectal lymph node(s)
N2	Metastasis in unilateral internal iliac and/or inguinal lymph node(s)
N3	Metastasis in internal iliac and perirectal lymph nodes and/or bilateral internal iliac and/or bilateral inguinal lymph nodes
Distant metastasis (M)	
M0	No distant metastasis
M1	Distant metastasis

MRI findings correlate well with physical findings concerning tumor size and therefore T stage whereas the infiltration of adjacent organs is often clinically underestimated. Extramural neoplastic spread may involve the sphincter complex muscles (external sphincter, levator ani and puborectalis) and most commonly occurs towards the anterior urogenital triangle, with possible involvement of the vagina, urethra, or bladder. Sometimes, the tumor may also extend laterally to invade the ischioanal fossa, superiorly to the rectum and mesorectal compartment or inferiorly to the skin and subcutaneous planes of the perianal region [1]. In such instances, T2-hyperintense solid tissue is seen encasing the lower signal intensity skeletal muscles, isointense structures such as the vagina, prostate, and urethra, or hyperintense fat in the ischiorectal and subcutaneous spaces [2, 7].

Imaging, particularly with MRI, also proves useful to differentiate anal carcinoma from other uncommon lesions arising inferior to the pelvic diaphragm, between the pubic symphysis and the coccyx, that usually manifest with similar symptoms and swelling or a mass. The differential diagnosis includes a wide spectrum of benign and malignant abnormalities such as pilonidal sinus diseases, cysts of Gartner duct or Bartolini gland, tailgut cysts, soft-tissue neoplasms (angiomyxoma, sacrococcygeal teratoma, liposarcoma, solitary fibrous tumor), urethral cancer, lymphoma, or metastases from colorectal, bladder, or prostatic primary cancer [3, 10].

Standard treatment for anal carcinoma currently relies on combined chemo- and radiotherapy, yielding satisfactory results with an overall patient survival of 70–80% after 5 years. Surgery with abdominoperineal resection is reserved for treatment failure with persistent or recurrent tumors [1, 3].

After radiochemotherapy, MRI provides confident assessment of the therapeutic response due to the intrinsic reproducibility of this modality. Findings indicative of a positive response include size reduction and diminished T2 signal intensity of the treated tumor (Fig. 26.2) [1, 2, 7]. Stability in size and signal intensity of any residual abnormality visible at MRI in the site of the treated lesion 1 year after therapy is strongly associated with a favorable outcome [1]. Conversely, persistent and locally recurrent tumors often have an aggressive behavior, with possible extensive involvement of the adjacent organs and pelvic bony structures, and a marked tendency for lymphatic dissemination [2].

References

1. Koh DM, Dzik-Jurasz A, O'Neill B, et al (2008) Pelvic phased-array MR imaging of anal carcinoma before and after chemoradiation. Br J Radiol 81:91-98
2. Parikh J, Shaw A, Grant LA, et al (2011) Anal carcinomas: the role of endoanal ultrasound and magnetic resonance imaging in staging, response evaluation and follow-up. Eur Radiol 21:776-785
3. Tappouni RF, Sarwani NI, Tice JG, et al (2011) Imaging of unusual perineal masses. AJR Am J Roentgenol 196:W412-420
4. Ky A, Sohn N, Weinstein MA, et al (1998) Carcinoma arising in anorectal fistulas of Crohn's disease. Dis Colon Rectum 41:992-996

5. Sjodahl RI, Myrelid P, Soderholm JD (2003) Anal and rectal cancer in Crohn's disease. Colorectal Dis 5:490-495
6. Devon KM, Brown CJ, Burnstein M, et al (2009) Cancer of the anus complicating perianal Crohn's disease. Dis Colon Rectum 52:211-216
7. Roach SC, Hulse PA, Moulding FJ, et al (2005) Magnetic resonance imaging of anal cancer. Clin Radiol 60:1111-1119
8. Glynne-Jones R, Northover JM, Cervantes A (2010) Anal cancer: ESMO Clinical Practice Guidelines for diagnosis, treatment and follow-up. Ann Oncol 21 Suppl 5:v87-92
9. Otto SD, Lee L, Buhr HJ, et al (2009) Staging anal cancer: prospective comparison of transanal endoscopic ultrasound and magnetic resonance imaging. J Gastrointest Surg 13:1292-1298
10. Hoeffel C, Crema MD, Azizi L, et al (2007) Magnetic resonance imaging of the ischiorectal fossa: spectrum of disease. J Comput Assist Tomogr 31:251-257

Rare Diseases

27

Massimo Tonolini

Hidradenitis suppurativa (HS) s a chronic inflammatory disease of the skin and subcutaneous tissues, occurring in apocrine-gland-bearing areas such as the axillae, inframammary regions, and perineum [1]. It is an uncommon, often debilitating disease with a chronic progressive course, including remissions and exacerbations. Usually diagnosed in young adults, HS is globally more frequent among females and blacks. Conversely, a perianal localization is more seen in men [2]. Poor hygiene has been suggested as a contributing factor in the onset of the disease. Currently, HS is considered as a disease caused by follicular occlusion rather than an inflammatory or infectious process of the apocrine glands, but its pathogenetic mechanisms are still unknown [3-5].

Clinically, patients with this rare condition present with tender subcutaneous nodules that spontaneously rupture or merge into painful, deep dermal abscesses, whereas advanced manifestations include fibrosis, ulceration, and the formation of extensive sinus tracts. Perianal HS is associated with more debilitating outcomes and is not unusually diagnosed in late stages due to social embarrassment and failure to seek medical treatment [2, 3]. The diagnosis of HS is mostly based on clinical evaluation. A classification system proposed by Hurley groups patients into three stages according to the presence and extent of cicatrization and sinuses. Since skin thickening and inflammation, induration of the subcutaneous tissues, abscesses, and fistulous tracts are nonspecific manifestations, perianal HS may thus mimic the presentation of other perianal inflammatory and infectious conditions, particularly cryptoglandular disease, Crohn's disease, as well as dermatological and sexually transmitted diseases [1].

In the past, the treatment of HS consisted of long-term antibiotics, antiandrogens, and surgery; recently, tumor necrosis factor inhibitors (anti-TNF)

M. Tonolini (✉)
Radiology Department, Luigi Sacco University Hospital
Milan, Italy
e-mail: mtonolini@sirm.org

M.Tonolini and G. Maconi (eds.), *Imaging of Perianal Inflammatory Diseases*,
DOI: 10.1007/978-88-470-2847-0_27, © Springer-Verlag Italia 2013

have introduced a promising therapeutic option for patients with this difficult disease. However, in patients with multiple interconnected sinus tracts and abscesses, only surgery can adequately address symptoms, and wide excision of all affected tissue is the most effective treatment. Unfortunately, HS shows a high recurrence rate even in surgically treated patients [1, 2].

Ultrasound may be useful for preliminary imaging assessment and in the exclusion of abnormalities involving scrotal sac contents but it does not allow a panoramic view of the entire perineal district, thus preventing an accurate assessment of disease extent.

Inflammatory changes and abscesses are easily identified by MRI, particularly with fat-suppression techniques and intravenous contrast; yet, to date, there have been few reports on the MRI findings in HS. The lesions are chronic and confined to superficial structures, with a typical symmetric distribution involving the pubis and scrotum, perineum, and medial aspects of the thighs. The usually prominent thickening of the skin and the indurated subcutaneous tissues show low signal intensity on T1-weighted images and high signal intensity on T2-weighted and STIR sequences, consistent with tissue edema and inflammation. Multiple but small fluid collections with peripheral enhancement after intravenous contrast administration corresponding to subcutaneous abscesses are usually present, along with sinus tracts and fistulas (Fig. 27.1) [6].

Almost invariably, there is no communication with the pelvic organs, including the bladder, urethra, rectum or anus; enlarged lymph nodes are present in inguinal regions [6].

MRI represents a highly valuable tool for the accurate diagnosis and assessment of disease extension and severity, as it clearly describes the anatomy of the affected area and facilitates planning of the surgical approach, which in turn reduce the risk of incomplete excision and recurrence.

Besides perianal fistulas and abscesses, the most important differential diagnosis is Fournier's gangrene (FG), an acute necrotizing fasciitis involving the genital, perineal, and perianal regions. FG is usually diagnosed in diabetics or immunodepressed patients and has a severe clinical presentation as well as a high mortality rate. Since FG represents a true surgical emergency, radiologic imaging should be followed by a prompt diagnostic confirmation. On plain radiographs, abnormal gas collections may be recognized in the involved areas whereas at ultrasound thickened superficial planes show strong hyperechogenicity with distal shadowing related to subcutaneous emphysema. In most cases, CT is the mainstay imaging modality as it provides a quick and comprehensive visualization of FG-related abnormalities, including skin involvement, subcutaneous and fascial thickening in the affected regions, abscess-like fluid structures with peripheral enhancement, and extensive gas collections (Fig. 27.2) [7, 8].

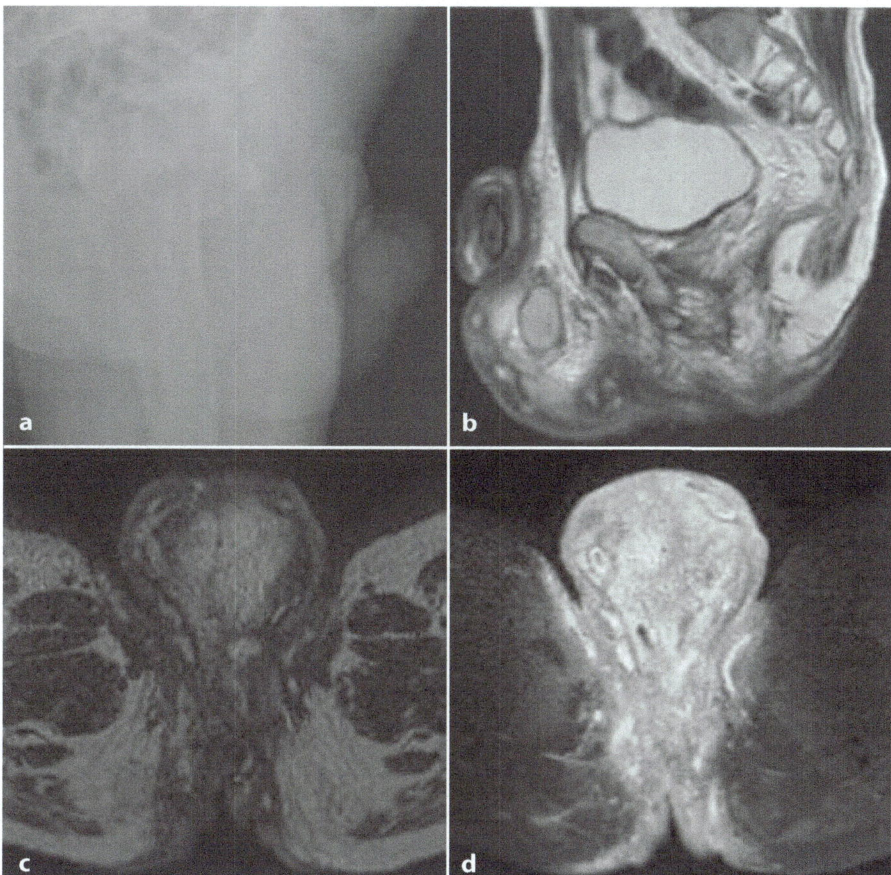

Fig. 27.1 A 51-year-old male with chronic HCV-related liver disease who presented with painful, massive swelling and inflammation of the perineum, scrotum, and penis that had progressively increased in recent months. The latero-lateral radiograph (**a**) documents marked swelling of the scrotum and penis without detectable gas collections, thus excluding Fournier's gangrene. Sagittal (**b**) and axial (**c**) T2-weighted images and the contrast-enhanced axial fat-suppressed T1-weighted (**d**) images show marked thickening of the skin and subcutaneous planes of the medial aspect of the thighs, perineal region, penis, and scrotum, all of which are involved by acute inflammation, with small pus collections. Hidradenitis suppurativa was diagnosed and the patient underwent antibiotic therapy, surgical incision, and drainage and curettage of the multiple scrotal abscesses

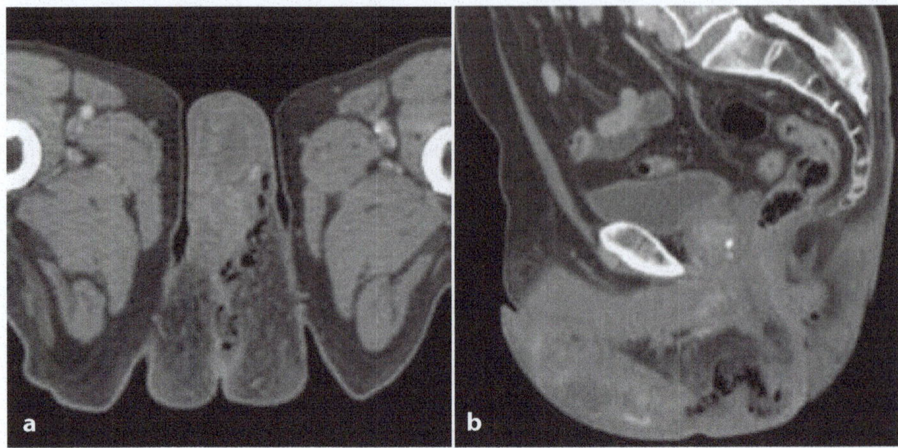

Fig. 27.2 A 67-year-old diabetic male who presented with perineal pain and swelling. Following urologic consultation, urgent CT was requested. Axial (**a**) and sagittal-reformatted (**b**) contrast-enhanced CT images show mixed fluid and air collections extending from the anal region ventrally towards the scrotum. The imaging diagnosis of Fournier's gangrene (probably secondary to an untreated urogenital infection) was confirmed during surgical intervention

References

1. Mortimer PS, Lunniss PJ (2000) Hidradenitis suppurativa. J R Soc Med 93:420-422
2. Anderson BB, Cadogan CA, Gangadharam D (1982) Hidradenitis suppurativa of the perineum, scrotum, and gluteal area: presentation, complications, and treatment. J Natl Med Assoc 74:999-1003
3. Alikhan A, Lynch PJ, Eisen DB (2009) Hidradenitis suppurativa: a comprehensive review. J Am Acad Dermatol 60:539-561; quiz 562-533
4. Kurzen H, Kurokawa I, Jemec GB, et al. (2008) What causes hidradenitis suppurativa? Exp Dermatol 17:455-456; discussion 457-472
5. Parks RW, Parks TG (1997) Pathogenesis, clinical features and management of hidradenitis suppurativa. Ann R Coll Surg Engl 79:83-89
6. Kelly AM, Cronin P (2005) MRI features of hidradenitis suppurativa and review of the literature. AJR Am J Roentgenol 185:1201-1204
7. Pavlica P, Barozzi L (2001) Imaging of the acute scrotum. Eur Radiol 11:220-228.
8. Piedra T, Ruiz E, Gonzalez FJ, et al (2006) Fournier's gangrene: a radiologic emergency. Abdom Imaging 31:500-502

Artifacts and Pitfalls

28

Massimo Tonolini

As extensively discussed in previous chapters, MRI currently represents the imaging modality of choice to assess fistula tract topography and the possible presence of abscess collections, since it can identify active sepsis despite the absence of an external opening [1, 2]. However, to date, no studies have been published concerning the learning curve and the importance of the reader's experience in interpreting perianal MRI findings.

Uncertainty regarding the MRI examination and thus misinterpretation may occur with small, intersphincteric fistulous tracts due to the limited extent of the pathologic process compared to the spatial resolution allowed by the acquisition with external phased-array MR coils (Fig. 28.1). Similarly, the identification of clinically evident superficial fistulas often proves challenging on MRI because of their small caliber and length. Originating below the lower sphincteric margin, superficial fistulas are located very close to and are usually indistinguishable from the lower margin of the external anal sphincter [1]. Since they do not disrupt muscular tissue, neither superficial fistulas nor anovaginal tracts are included in the most widely adopted classifications. Simple anovaginal fistulas mostly consist of short, thin-walled, and collapsed tracts surrounded by adipose tissue and a venous plexus in the anovaginal septum. As our unpublished experience has confirmed (50% sensitivity for anovaginal fistulas without abscess collections), MRI is unreliable particularly in the absence of precise clinical suspicion (Fig. 28.2) [3].

A not infrequent source of interpretation error for the inexperienced radiologist involves the presence of veins running in the ischioanal spaces, which is not unusual but can they be misinterpreted as fistulas. Correct identification of these normal, enhancing structures should rely on their thin-walled, tortuous,

M. Tonolini (✉)
Radiology Department, Luigi Sacco University Hospital
Milan, Italy
e-mail: mtonolini@sirm.org

M.Tonolini and G. Maconi (eds.), *Imaging of Perianal Inflammatory Diseases*,
DOI: 10.1007/978-88-470-2847-0_28, © Springer-Verlag Italia 2013

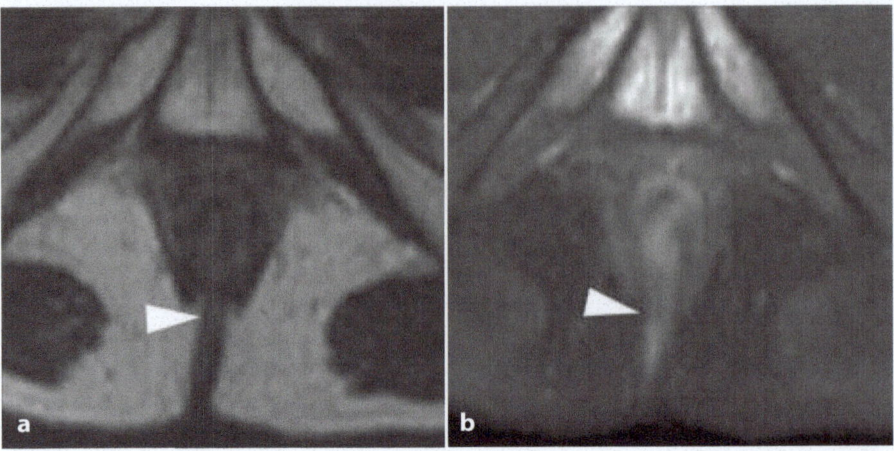

Fig. 28.1 A 46-year-old male patient with Crohn's disease. There is a very subtle posterior linear tract on the T2-weighted axial image (**a**), with linear enhancement after intravenous gadolinium as seen on the axial contrast-enhanced fat-saturated T1-weighted image (**b**). This active simple intersphincteric fistula was initially detected by means of transperineal ultrasound

and branching appearance, and on their usual symmetric presence on both sides (Fig. 28.3) [3].

Sometimes, the classification of perianal inflammatory disease on MRI studies according to the Parks' and St. James' University Hospital (SJUH) schemes may prove challenging for the radiologist, with a non-negligible interpretation uncertainty. Not unexpectedly, interobserver agreement has been reported to be significantly higher for the detection of abscesses and horseshoe fistulas than for simple tracts [1, 4]. In our experience, the MRI-based SJUH staging system is more easily adopted in everyday radiologic practice and we strongly suggest its application in reporting MRI examinations.

A fistulous external opening is not an issue at MRI, since its presence and draining status are always assessed clinically and are generally evident at surgical inspection. According to Goodsall's rule, a fistula having an external orifice situated behind the transverse anal line opens into the anal canal in the midline posteriorly [2].

Also, an internal fistulous opening, often situated along the dentate line, can be diagnostically very challenging if MRI is acquired using phased-array coils, but it is usually detected at surgical examination and/or proctoscopy. On MRI, the internal opening is usually obscured when abscess collections abut the anal canal; instead, it can usually be inferred from the course and orientation of the fistulous tract [4].

The crucial distinction between an intersphincteric vs. a transsphincteric inflammatory process relies on the identification of fistulous crossing through the external sphincter towards the ischioanal fat space [2]. Sometimes, uncer-

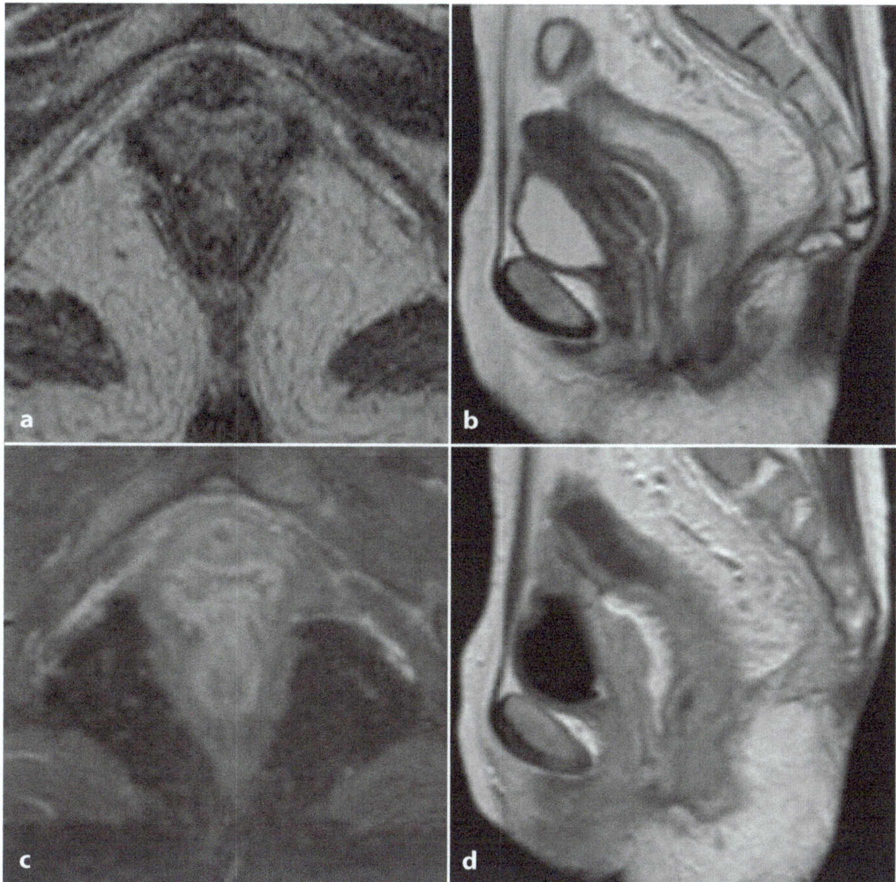

Fig. 28.2 A female patient with previously diagnosed Crohn's disease. On axial (**a**) and sagittal (**b**) T2-weighted images and on axial contrast-enhanced fat-saturated (**c**) and sagittal (**d**) T1-weighted images, there is midline obliteration of the normal, thin fat layer of the anovaginal septum by intermediate T2 signal intensity tissue with moderate enhancement. Correlation with symptoms and transperineal ultrasound allowed the diagnosis of a collapsed anovaginal fistula

tainty exists when healed fibrotic tracts must be differentiated from inactive fistulas that are still patent but not filled with fluid (Fig. 28.4) [2, 4].

There is no clear-cut definition regarding the minimum size of abscess collections. Variable cut-off values have been suggested, ranging from 3 mm to 1 cm. This has undoubtedly contributed to inconsistencies in radiologic reports since SJUH grade 2 and grade 4 perianal inflammations are distinguished from those of grade 1 and grade 3, respectively, by the presence of an abscess or a secondary tract [5]. Suprasphincteric vs. extrasphincteric (translevator) Parks' fistulas are not easily differentiated on MRI, but these two anatomically distinct

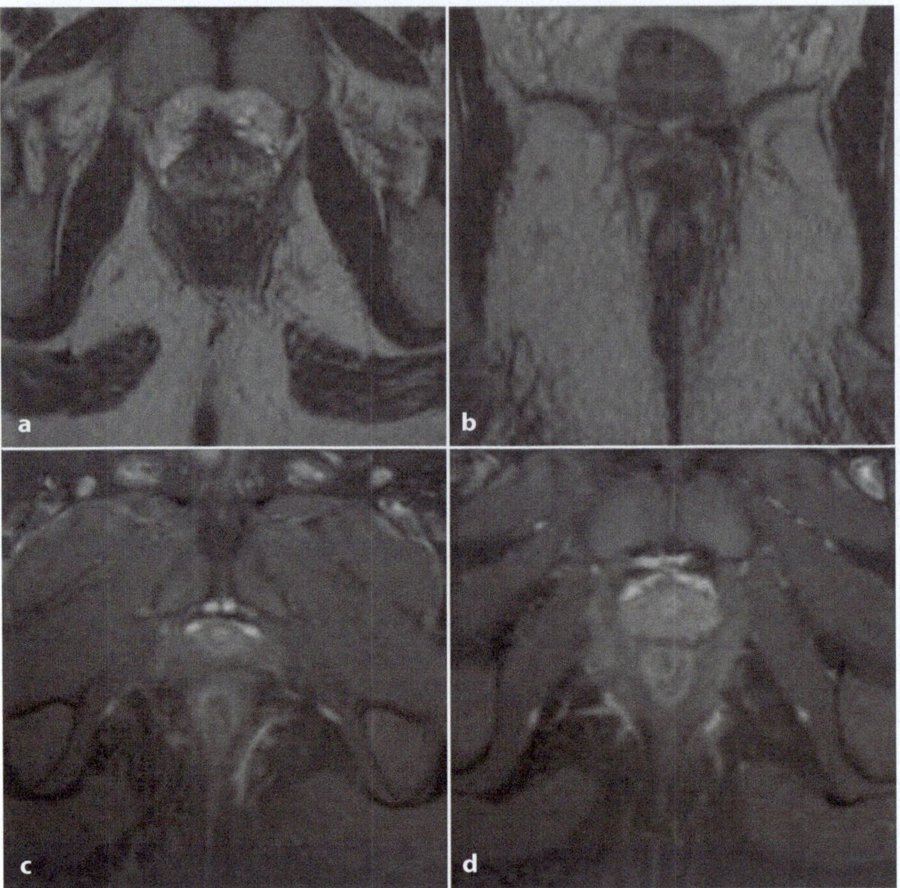

Fig. 28.3 Veins running symmetrically in the ischioanal fat spaces, seen as thin, linear structures with branching on axial (**a**) and coronal (**b**) T2-weighted images, enhancing after intravenous gadolinium administration on axial post-contrast fat-saturated (**c, d**) T1-weighted images. These findings did not correspond to clinical or transperineal ultrasound evidence of perianal inflammation and should not be mistaken for fistulas

lesions are grouped to form grade 5 of the SJUH classification. Furthermore, unilateral thickening of the levator ani muscle, which based on MRI criteria is suspicious for infectious involvement, may instead be reactive to the presence of an adjacent abscess collection below or above it [5].

When MRI is requested to reassess medically or surgically treated perianal inflammation, commonly persistent high T2-weighted signal intensity and positive contrast enhancement are observed even long after therapy-induced clinical healing, probably reflecting the unreliable imaging differentiation between persistently active sepsis and healing granulation tissue (Fig. 28.5) [6, 7].

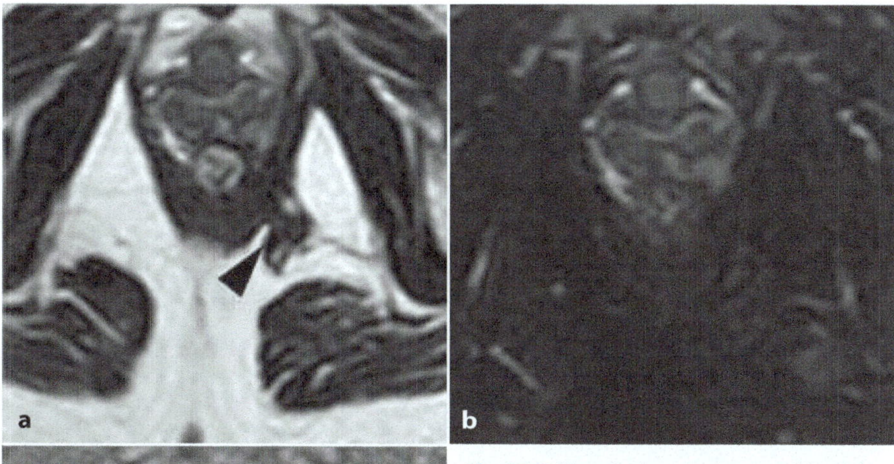

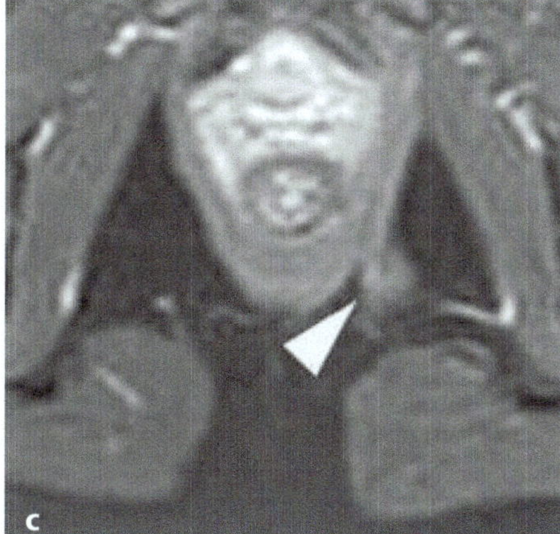

Fig. 28.4 Chronic (inactive) transsphincteric fistula. Axial T2-weighted (**a**) and STIR (**b**) images depict a simple fistula crossing the external sphincter and reaching the ischioanal fossa on the left side, with low signal intensity consistent with fibrosis. Minimal residual enhancement is seen after intravenous gadolinium administration on an axial contrast-enhanced fat-saturated T1-weighted image (**c**)

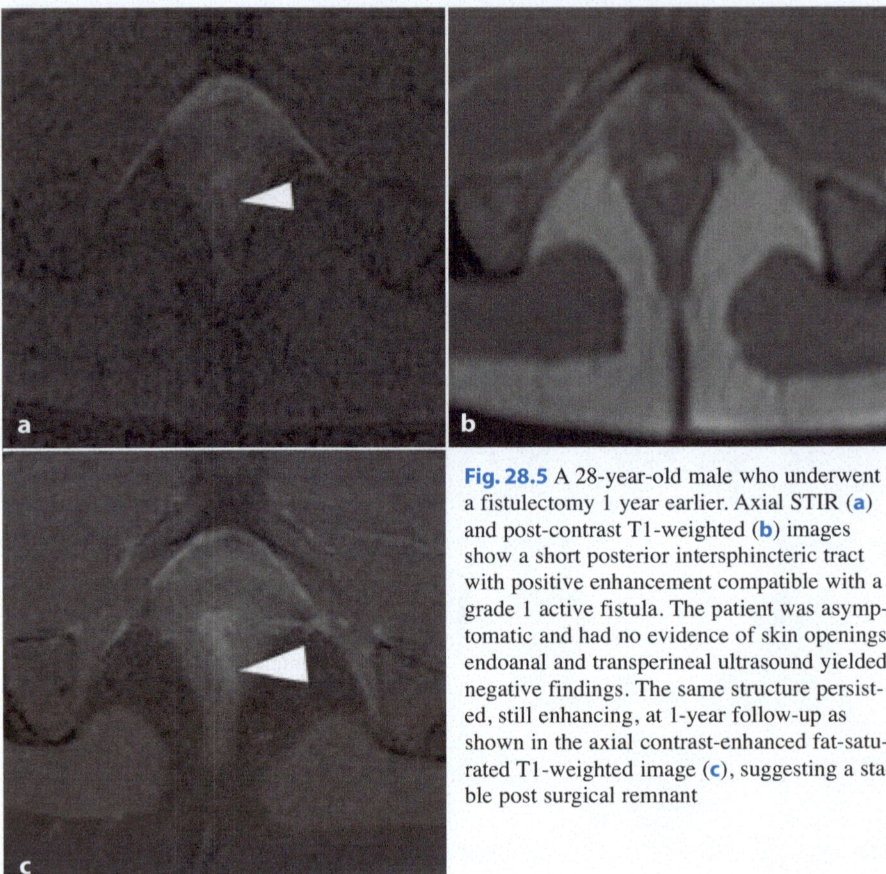

Fig. 28.5 A 28-year-old male who underwent a fistulectomy 1 year earlier. Axial STIR (**a**) and post-contrast T1-weighted (**b**) images show a short posterior intersphincteric tract with positive enhancement compatible with a grade 1 active fistula. The patient was asymptomatic and had no evidence of skin openings; endoanal and transperineal ultrasound yielded negative findings. The same structure persisted, still enhancing, at 1-year follow-up as shown in the axial contrast-enhanced fat-saturated T1-weighted image (**c**), suggesting a stable post surgical remnant

References

1. Szurowska E, Wypych J, Izycka-Swieszewska E (2007) Perianal fistulas in Crohn's disease: MRI diagnosis and surgical planning: MRI in fistulazing perianal Crohn's disease. Abdom Imaging 32:705-718
2. Maccioni F, Colaiacomo MC, Stasolla A, et al. (2002) Value of MRI performed with phased-array coil in the diagnosis and pre-operative classification of perianal and anal fistulas. Radiol Med 104:58-67
3. Horsthuis K, Stoker J (2004) MRI of perianal Crohn's disease. Am J Roent 183:1309-1315
4. Beets-Tan RG, Beets GL, van der Hoop AG, et al. (2001) Preoperative MR imaging of anal fistulas: Does it really help the surgeon? Radiology 218:75-84
5. Hussain SM, Outwater EK, Joekes EC, et al. (2000) Clinical and MR imaging features of cryptoglandular and Crohn's fistulas and abscesses. Abdom Imaging 25:67-74
6. Bell SJ, Halligan S, Windsor AC, et al. (2003) Response of fistulating Crohn's disease to infliximab treatment assessed by magnetic resonance imaging. Aliment Pharmacol Ther 17:387-393
7. Van Assche G, Vanbeckevoort D, Bielen D, et al. (2003) Magnetic resonance imaging of the effects of infliximab on perianal fistulizing Crohn's disease. Am J Gastroenterol 98:332-339

Techniques and Role of CT in Perianal Disease

29

Alba H. Norsa and Massimo Tonolini

29.1 Introduction

Cross-sectional imaging studies are an essential component in the assessment of perianal inflammatory disease, including its anatomic relationship with the anal sphincter complex, and in monitoring disease evolution following medical or surgical treatment [1]. In the 1980s and 1990s, CT was introduced to investigate the presence and extent of inflammatory changes in patients with Crohn's disease (CD). Careful interpretation of anatomic landmarks on thick-section axial images was necessary to distinguish supra- from infralevator compartment abscesses [2, 3].

Currently, MRI acquisition with phased-array coils is the modality of choice to identify and stage perianal fistulas and abscesses with high accuracy, allowing excellent visualization of anorectal and perineal structures and their abnormalities. The intrinsic advantages of MRI include multiplanarity, biological non-invasiveness, an excellent paramagnetic contrast safety profile, and high spatial and contrast resolution [4-6]. Therefore, most authors nowadays consider CT to be an obsolete technique in the assessment of perianal disease when MRI and endoanal/transperineal ultrasound are available [1].

Nonetheless, as a CT device has become standard in most hospitals of industrialized countries, urgent CT examinations are widely requested to investigate re-exacerbations or acute abdominal complications occurring in patients with CD. In this setting, CT allows the detection of variable-degree obstruction, perforation, internal fistulization, and abscess collections [7]. Furthermore, current multidetector scanners easily overcome most of the lim-

A.H. Norsa (✉)
Radiology Department, IGEA Clinic
Milan, Italy
e-mail: alba.norsa@gmail.com

M.Tonolini and G. Maconi (eds.), *Imaging of Perianal Inflammatory Diseases*,
DOI: 10.1007/978-88-470-2847-0_29, © Springer-Verlag Italia 2013

itations of axial CT based on their extremely fast acquisition and panoramic coverage of the entire abdomen and pelvis in a few seconds, with volumetric resolution and isotropic image reconstruction on arbitrary planes. Intravenous contrast injection during CT is recommended in most situations involving inflammatory bowel diseases (Fig. 29.1) [8].

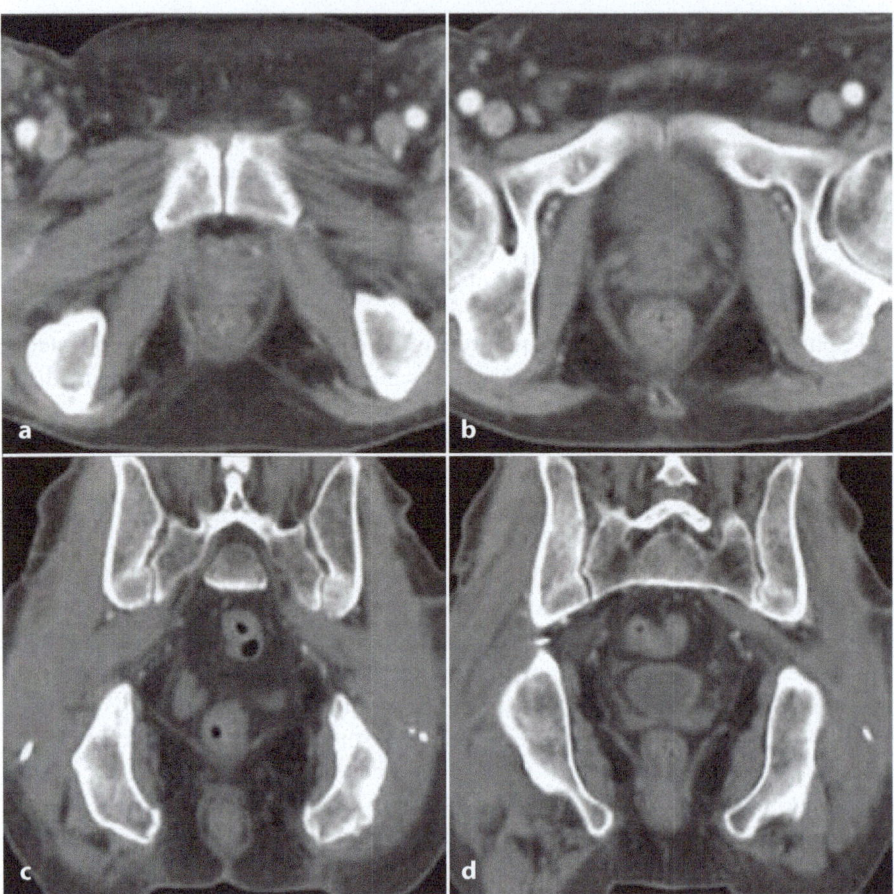

Fig. 29.1 A 55-year-old HIV-positive male patient with clinical suspicion of recurrent perianal infection following previous surgical treatment many years earlier. MRI was contraindicated because of poor patient cooperation and the presence of numerous metallic needles in both buttocks. Axial (**a**, **b**) and coronal-reformatted (**c**, **d**) images from pelvic contrast-enhanced CT provide adequate visualization of anorectal and perianal anatomic structures, without signs of abscess formation in the intersphincteric, supralevator, and ischioanal spaces

29.2 CT in the Evaluation of Perianal Disease

Perianal abscesses and fistulas that are filled by air or fluid can be identified on CT because of adequate contrast between their hypodense contents and the enhancing, inflamed granulation tissue present in the walls. Intrinsic CT contrast resolution limits the differentiation between different soft-tissue structures such as the pelvic muscles, active inflammatory changes, and fibrotic scar tissue (Fig. 29.2) [2, 5, 9]. Multidetector CT acquisition including routine multiplanar reconstructions enables the detection of inflammatory changes and their relationships to the anal sphincter complex and ischioanal spaces, with a relia-

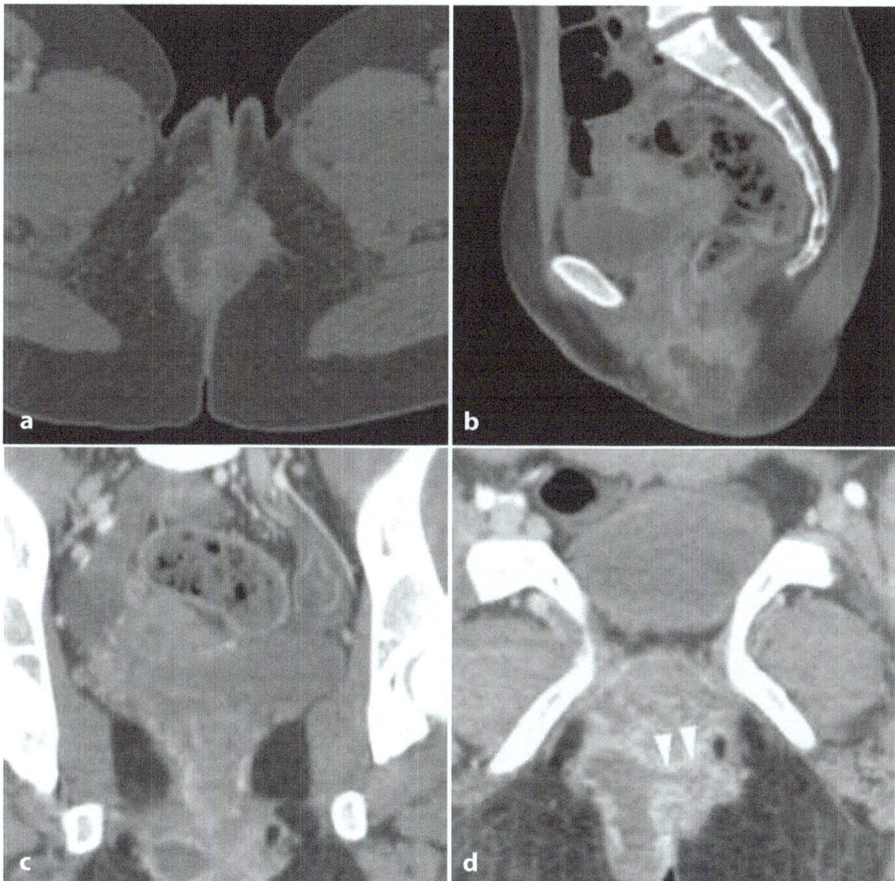

Fig. 29.2 A 27-year-old female patient with ulcerative colitis. A distal perineal abscess was detected clinically and confirmed by transperineal ultrasound. Axial (**a**), sagittal (**b**), and coronal (**c**) reformatted images from a contrast-enhanced volumetric MDCT acquisition visualize the entire extent of the right-sided abscess collection along three planes. The oblique reformation (**d**) identifies the fistulous tract with a small gas bubble, giving rise to the abscess (*arrowheads*)

bility approaching that of MRI (Figs. 29.1, 29.2). The lower sensitivity (77%) of CT for the detection of perianal abscesses in immunosuppressed patients has been reported, probably because of a poor inflammatory response. In these patients, it is difficult to detect enhancement corresponding to active inflammation [9]. Notably, a significant limitation persists in the assessment of the thin, normal, fat-containing anovaginal and intersphincteric spaces [2, 3, 5].

Nonetheless, the main disadvantage of CT remains its dependence on ionizing radiation. Chronic inflammatory bowel diseases mostly affect young people, whose life expectancy will nonetheless be normal but with frequent exacerbations or complications, leading to a need for repeated diagnostic imaging studies. Therefore, patients and physicians are justifiably concerned about radiation over-exposure, with its associated increased risk of malignancy. Recently, a retrospective study addressing the total effective dose of ionizing radiation in patients with inflammatory bowel diseases over a 5-year period determined higher cumulative radiation exposure in patients with CD than in those with ulcerative colitis; some patients (7%) had been exposed to very high radiation levels (>50 mSv), the vast majority during CT scans [10]. Therefore, the frequent need for imaging studies contraindicates the use of diagnostic imaging with ionizing radiation in patients with CD; instead, ultrasound and MRI are the preferred imaging modalities [1, 8, 9].

In patients with CD who undergo elective (such as CT-enteroclysis or CT-enterography) or urgent MDCT acquisitions, anatomic coverage should be extended to include the entire perianal and genital region, and coronal plane reconstructions routinely performed. Abscess involvement at the level of or above the levator ani muscles is identifiable on coronal images. Inhomogeneity, abnormal density, or enhancement involving the ischioanal fat spaces indicates the presence of transsphincteric inflammation, to be further investigated with MRI (Figs. 29.3, 29.4) [2, 3, 9].

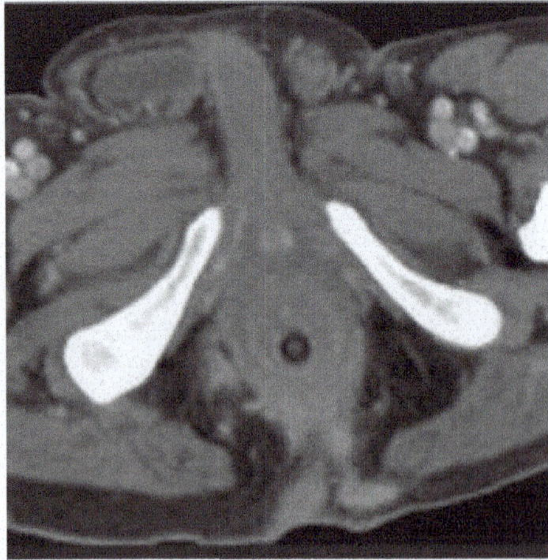

Fig. 29.3 A 60-year-old male with elevated serum tumor markers who underwent abdominopelvic CT with a retrograde water enema (note rectal probe in place) to investigate bowel inflammation. This caudalmost image shows an enhancing fistulous tract crossing the left ischioanal fossa

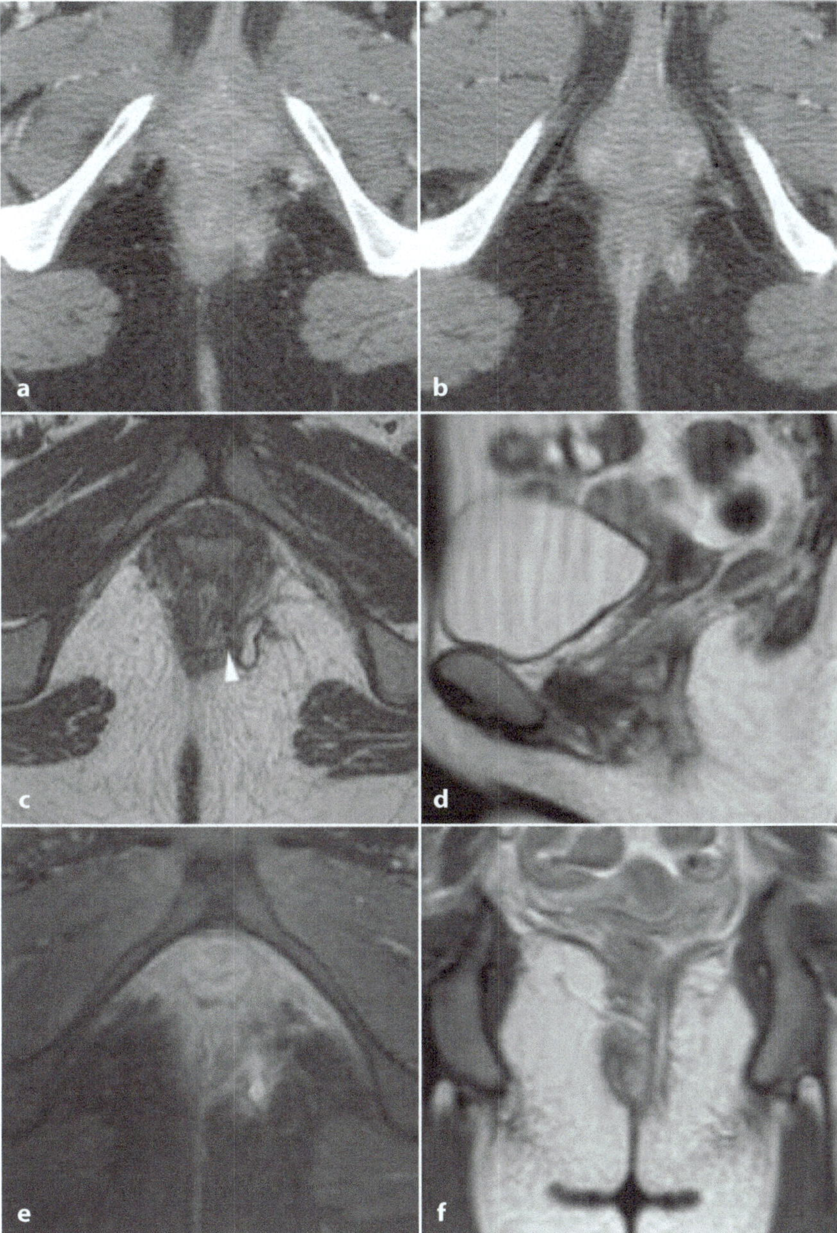

Fig. 29.4 A 21-year-old female with Crohn's disease who underwent urgent contrast-enhanced multidetector CT during an acute abdominal exacerbation. The caudalmost CT images (**a**, **b**) show a left-sided, enhancing, transsphincteric fistula, to be further investigated with MRI. Axial (**c**) and sagittal (**d**) T2-weighted images and post-contrast fat-suppressed axial (**e**) and coronal (**f**) T1-weighted images better depict the fluid-containing, vertically oriented fistula, including its internal opening (*arrowhead* in c), which strongly enhances after intravenous contrast

In conclusion, multidetector CT with intravenous contrast medium provides a sufficiently accurate assessment of perianal inflammatory changes in CD patients and may prove useful when MRI is not available or contraindicated, such as in patients with claustrophobia, cardiac pacemakers, or metallic foreign bodies. However, the non-negligible radiation dose involved should limit the use of CT, particularly in young patients and in those in whom repeated studies are necessary [3, 5, 10].

References

1. Ziech M, Felt-Bersma R, Stoker J (2009) Imaging of perianal fistulas. Clin Gastroenterol Hepatol 7:1037-1045
2. Guillaumin E, Jeffrey RB, Jr., Shea WJ, et al (1986) Perirectal inflammatory disease: CT findings. Radiology 161:153-157
3. Halligan S, Stoker J (2006) Imaging of fistula in ano. Radiology 239:18-33
4. Torkzad MR, U. K (2011) MRI for assessment of anal fistula. Insights Imaging 1:62-71
5. Szurowska E, Wypych J, Izycka-Swieszewska E (2007) Perianal fistulas in Crohn's disease: MRI diagnosis and surgical planning : MRI in fistulazing perianal Crohn's disease. Abdom Imaging 32:705-718
6. Maccioni F, Colaiacomo MC, Stasolla A, et al (2002) Value of MRI performed with phased-array coil in the diagnosis and pre-operative classification of perianal and anal fistulas. Radiol Med 104:58-67
7. Cellini C, Safar B, Fleshman J (2010) Surgical management of pyogenic complications of Crohn's disease. Inflamm Bowel Dis 16:512-517
8. Laniado M, Makowiec F, Dammann F, et al (1997) Perianal complications of Crohn disease: MR imaging findings. Eur Radiol 7:1035-1042
9. Caliste X, Nazir S, Goode T, et al (2011) Sensitivity of computed tomography in detection of perirectal abscess. Am Surg 77:166-168
10. Kroeker KI, Lam S, Birchall I, et al (2011) Patients with IBD are exposed to high levels of ionizing radiation through CT scan diagnostic imaging: a five-year study. J Clin Gastroenterol 45:34-39

Integration of Diagnostic Modalities and Diagnostic Algorithms

30

Cristina Bezzio and Giovanni Maconi

30.1 Introduction

The management of patients with perianal disease, and in particular those with perianal fistula, depends on the careful evaluation of the clinical history, the findings of the physical examination, and an assessment of intestinal diseases and perianal lesions (Fig. 30.1) [1]. These steps are mandatory to plan proper treatment, which may be medical, surgical, or, as is often the case, a combination of the two. Medical therapy mainly consists of antibiotics, anti-tumor necrosis factor alpha, and immunosuppressants, whilst in surgical treatment fistulotomy, fistulectomy, seton placement, endorectal advancement flaps, fecal diversion, and proctocolectomy are the most common procedures.

The treatment of perianal fistulas depends mainly on the nature of the lesion, whether cryptogenetic or Crohn's related, and on its classification. The latter takes into account several aspects, such as the anatomical site of the internal opening, the course of the fistula in relation to the anal sphincters, and in particular the presence of extensions, branches, and perianal abscesses.

The main diagnostic tools currently used to classify perianal fistulas are transanal ultrasound, magnetic resonance imaging (MRI), exam under anesthesia (EUA), and trans-perineal ultrasound. However, sometimes these procedures are contraindicated or not available; moreover, their accuracy is less than 100%. A recent meta-analysis assessed the accuracy of transanal ultrasound and MRI for detecting perianal fistula, showing that the sensitivity of these methods was comparable and high (87% for each one) and that the specificity of MRI was higher than that of transanal ultrasound (63% vs. 43%).

G. Maconi (✉)
Gastroenterology Unit, Department of Biomedical and Clinical Sciences
Luigi Sacco University Hospital
Milan, Italy
e-mail: giovanni.maconi@unimi.it

M.Tonolini and G. Maconi (eds.), *Imaging of Perianal Inflammatory Diseases*,
DOI: 10.1007/978-88-470-2847-0_30, © Springer-Verlag Italia 2013

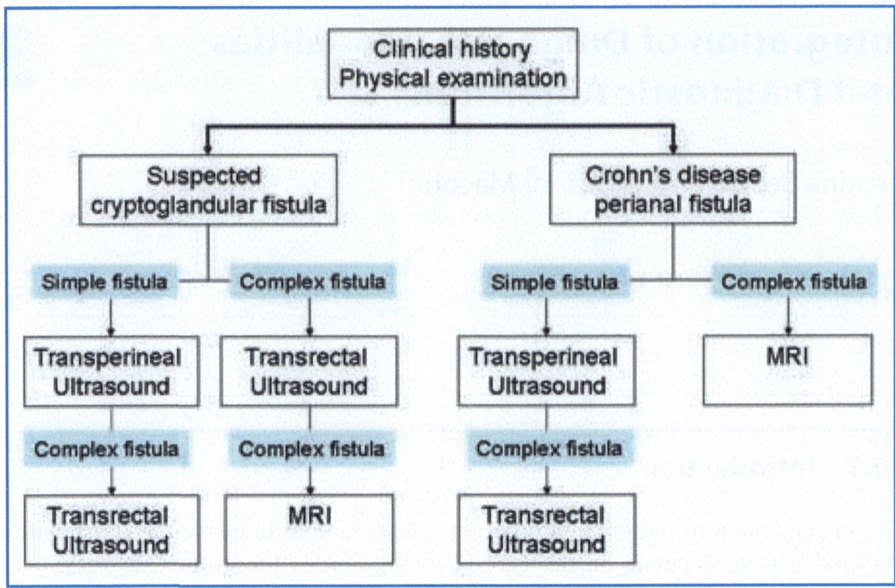

Figure 30.1 Suggested flowchart for the use of imaging techniques in patients with perianal fistulas. Patients with suspected perianal fistulas may be stratified based on the presence or absence of Crohn's disease. Those with a suspected fistula of cryptoglandular origin may benefit from perianal ultrasound as the initial imaging examination. In patients in whom the clinical diagnosis of simple fistula has been confirmed, the diagnostic work-up may be stopped, whilst in those with complex fistulas the recommended approach consists of further investigations by means of transanal ultrasound (with or without peroxide fistulography), MRI, or both before exam under anesthesia and/or surgical treatment

However, both specificity values are considered diagnostically poor, especially considering the heterogeneity between studies of the two procedures [2].

Missed lesions and false-positive results are also possible with simple surgical digital examination and even with EUA. While the former results in the incorrect assessment of primary tracts and abscesses in 40–60% of cases [3], the latter, even when performed by experts, may misclassify up to 10% of perianal fistulas [4]. These considerations should be taken into account in the planning of medical and surgical treatment, given that an inaccurate diagnosis may lead to disease progression, with an increased risk of recurrence, on the one hand, as well as to inappropriate surgery, with irreversible functional consequences on the other. Consequently, the correct use of imaging procedures, their appropriate combination, and the cooperation of radiologists, surgeons, and gastroenterologists are crucial for the successful treatment of perianal fistulas and the prevention of their recurrence.

30.2 Perianal Fistulas Classifications

To correctly plan treatment, the classification of perianal fistulas should be clearly interpretable by the involved surgeons and gastroenterologists. The most commonly and widely used classification system, that of Parks, dates from 1976 [5]. The Parks criteria rely on an anatomically precise system in which the external anal sphincter is the central reference point. Five types of perianal fistulas are therefore described: (a) intersphincteric fistula, characterized by a primary tract that courses in the intersphincteric space without penetrating (<30%) the external sphincter; (b) trans-sphincteric fistula, which traverses the external sphincter and passes into the ischioanal fossa, below the level of the puborectalis muscle; (c) suprasphincteric fistula, which travels within the intersphincteric plane superior to the puborectalis before penetrating the levator musculature to course within the ischiorectal and ischioanal fossae; (d) extrasphincteric fistula, which courses within the ischioanal fossa and penetrates the levator musculature without traversing either the internal or the external sphincters, instead opening directly into the rectum; and (e) superficial fistula.

However, these criteria have their limitations because they do not consider relevant information on perianal disease, such as the presence or absence of macroscopic rectal inflammation, co-existing perianal abscesses, or fistulous connection to other structures such as the bladder, vagina, or anal strictures, which may affect the choice of treatment as well as patient outcome. To overcome this deficit, an American Gastroenterological Association technical review panel on perianal Crohn's disease developed a simplified but more clinically relevant approach to classifying fistulas [6], describing them as either simple or complex. A simple fistula is a superficial, intersphincteric, or low trans-sphincteric fistula with only a single opening and not associated with an abscess and/or not connected to an adjacent structure such as the vagina or bladder. A complex fistula involves more of the anal sphincter (i.e., high trans-sphincteric, extrasphincteric or suprasphincteric), has multiple openings, horseshoeing (crossing the midline either anteriorly or posteriorly), an association with a perianal abscess, and/or a connection to an adjacent structure such as the vagina or bladder [6]

Patients with complex fistulas are at increased risk for incontinence following aggressive surgical intervention. They also have a reduced rate of fistula healing and greater likelihood of recurrence.

Other perianal disease classification systems and scores, such as the Cardiff classification and perianal disease activity index (PDAI), are rather complex; accordingly, their acceptance and use in clinical practice have been limited [7, 8].

Irrespective of the system employed to classify perianal fistula, an accurate description of the fistulous tracts is of utmost importance. The presence of branching or horseshoeing (crossing the midline anteriorly or posteriorly) and its location (intersphincteric, infralevator, supralevator) must be noted since the presence of either one may change the surgical management [9].

30.3 Comparison of Diagnostic Imaging Techniques in Perianal Fistulas

The choice of the imaging technique for the detection and characterization of perianal disease is currently based upon several factors: local availability and expertise, cost of the procedure, the particular features of the perianal disease, and the age of the patient as well as the disease duration. In some instances, the use of at least two modalities may be necessary; this is often the case in patients with recurrent or complicated perianal disease [10].

Ideally, patients without well known intestinal inflammatory disease in whom fistula-in-ano is suspected should, after the initial clinical history and physical and digital anorectal examinations, undergo transperineal ultrasound in order to confirm the diagnosis. This method is widely and promptly available, inexpensive, and according to the literature data sufficiently accurate both in confirming a perianal fistula and in classifying its type. Complex perianal fistula initially suspected at digital examination or assessed by preliminary trans-perineal ultrasound prior to EUA or surgical treatment should be assessed by transanal ultrasound, MRI, or both, according to the disease complexity and the surgeon's discretion (Fig. 30.1)

Table 1 provides a comparison between the proposed tests for the diagnosis and characterization of perianal fistulas in Crohn's disease. Transanal ultrasound, trans-perineal ultrasound and MRI are able to characterize perianal fistulas with an overall high level of accuracy, but with variable cost and invasiveness.

30.4 Diagnostic Algorithms

30.4.1 American Gastroenterological Association

According to the American Gastroenterological Association [6], the appropriate medical or surgical therapy should be initially planned based on the classification of perianal disease as simple or complex.

The diagnosis of simple fistulas and complex perianal disease by digital examination and rectosigmoidoscopy may be sufficient in those patients in whom medical therapy is the initial treatment strategy. However, in patients with suspected septic complications such as abscesses and in those with recurrent fistulas, other imaging modalities should be used to diagnose and classify Crohn's perianal fistulas, including EUA, pelvic MRI, and transanal ultrasound. In fact, it has been shown that only the combination of more than one diagnostic modality is able to reach an accuracy of 100% in the detection of fistulas and their complications. Therefore, additional diagnostic evaluation by EUA and either transanal ultrasound or MRI is indicated in patients with pain, fluctuation, or stricture as determined on digital rectal examination and in

Table 30.1 Comparison of the features of transperineal ultrasound, transanal ultrasound, and magnetic resonance imaging in the evaluation of perianal fistulas

Features	Transanal ultrasound	MRI	Transperineal ultrasound
Patient comfort	Quicker (5–10 min) examination Endoanal probe	Longer (45 min) examination No endoanal coil required Claustrophobia may be a problem	Quicker (5–10 min) No discomfort
Expense	Less expensive	More expensive	Less expensive
Characterization of the primary tract	Excellent	Excellent	Excellent
Characterization of the secondary tract	Excellent within the sphincter complex Limited if the tract extends far from the anal canal	Excellent	Good within the sphincter complex Limited if tracts extend far from the perianal skin
Identification of abscesses	Excellent within sphincter complex Limited if abscesses are distant from the anal canal	Excellent	Good within the sphincter complex Limited if abscesses are distant from the perianal skin
Evaluation of supralevator or pelvic disease	Limited, due to field of view considerations	Excellent	Limited, due to field of view considerations
Evaluation of tract patency	Excellent (when fistulography is performed)	Limited if the tract has collapsed	Excellent (when fistulography is performed)
Availability	Depends on local expertise Equipment usually available	Depends on local expertise Equipment not always available	Depends on local expertise Equipment widely available

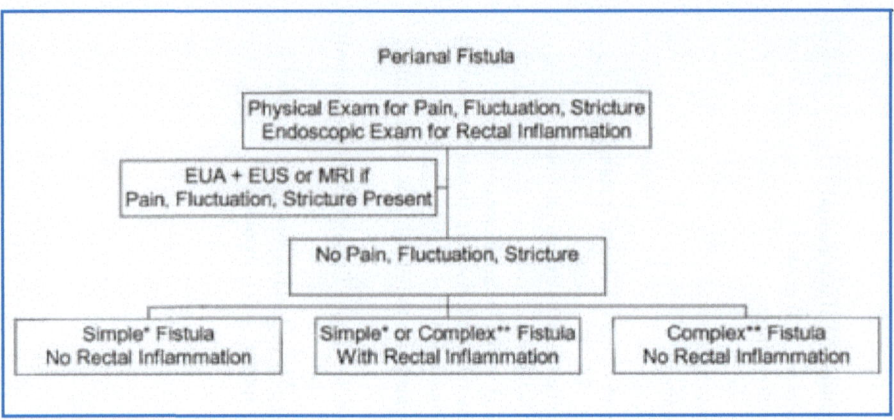

Figure 30.2 Diagnostic algorithm according to the AGA [6] for patients with Crohn's disease and perianal fistulas

and therapeutic relevance. In fact, anecdotal experience indicates that the treatment of fistulae is unsuccessful without treatment of the underlying active disease [3, 12].

EUA is the gold standard but only when performed by an experienced surgeon. If an abscess is present or suspected, prompt EUA, including drainage, is the procedure of choice to prevent the destructive effective of undrained sepsis. The procedure should not be delayed until an MRI has been performed, unless the scan is immediately available. Transanal ultrasound is accurate when conducted by experts and in conjunction with hydrogen peroxide enhancement. It provides a valid alternative to MRI. Fistulography is no longer recommended.

30.4.3 American Society of Colon and Rectal Surgeons

The Standards Practice Task Force of the American Society of Colon and Rectal Surgeons [13], composed of members with well-known expertise in the specialty of colon and rectal surgery, recently published practice guidelines for the management of abscess and fistula-in-ano. According to those guidelines, in the initial evaluation of perianal abscess and fistula-in-ano a disease-specific history should be obtained and a physical examination performed, both emphasizing symptoms, risk factors, location, and the presence of secondary cellulitis or fistula-in-ano. The task force stressed the importance of distinguishing anorectal abscess from other perianal suppurative processes (e.g., hidradenitis suppurativa, infected skin furuncles, and infectious diseases such as tuberculosis, syphilis, and actinomycosis). In addition, features suggestive of Crohn's disease, including large skin tags or multiple fistulas, should be noted as they require a more detailed workup and, potentially, additional medical therapy.

Palpation of the perianal area, digital rectal examination, and careful probing of the tract(s) are suggested to define the presence and anatomy of the fistula. Anoscopy and sigmoidoscopy are recommended to visualize the internal opening of the fistula and other mucosal abnormalities such as proctitis secondary to Crohn's disease.

Imaging studies including fistulography, transanal ultrasound, computed tomography (CT) scan, and MRI may be considered in selected patients to help define the anatomy of an anorectal abscess or fistula-in-ano and to guide management. Although both conditions can most commonly be diagnosed and managed on the basis of clinical findings alone, and the vast majority of fistulas do not require imaging, in patients with complex tracts or recurrent disease imaging studies can provide valuable information.

Among the diagnostic tests, fistulography has, as mentioned above, been abandoned, due to its low accuracy. Transanal ultrasound, however, is considered very effective for characterizing anorectal abscess and fistulas and in identifying horseshoe abscess extensions, especially if this modality is combined with 3-dimensional ultrasound techniques that include hydrogen peroxide injection.

CT scan and MRI are also useful for patients with complex suppurative anorectal conditions, particularly in the identification of supralevator abscesses, and in patients with Crohn's disease.

References

1. Koutroubakis IE (2007) The patient with persistent perianal fistulae. Best Pract Res Clin Gastroenterol 21:503-18
2. Siddiqui MR, Ashrafian H, Tozer P, et al (2012) A diagnostic accuracy meta-analysis of endoanal ultrasound and MRI for perianal fistula assessment. Dis Colon Rectum 55:576-85.
3. Buchanan GN, Halligan S, Bartram CI, et al (2004) Clinical examination, endosonography, and MR imaging in preoperative assessment of fistula in ano: comparison with outcome-based reference standard. Radiology 233:674-81
4. Schwartz DA, Loftus EV, Tremaine WJ, et al (2002) The natural history of fistulizing Crohn's disease in Olmsted County, Minnesota. Gastroenterology 122:875–80
5. Parks AG, Gordon PH, Hardcastle JD (1976) A classification of fistulain-ano. Br J Surg 63:1–12.
6. American Gastroenterological Association Clinical Practice Committee (2003) American Gastroenterological Association medical position statement: perianal Crohn's disease. Gastroenterology 125:1503–7.
7. Alexander-Williams J, Hellers G, Hughes LE, Minervini S, Speranza V (1992) Classification of perianal Crohn's disease. Gastroenterol Int 5:216–20
8. Pikarsky AJ, Gervaz P, Wexner SD (2002) Perianal Crohn disease: a new scoring system to evaluate and predict outcome of surgical intervention. Arch Surg 137:774–7
9. Halligan S, Stoker J (2006) Imaging of fistula in ano. Radiology 239:18-33

10. Sun MR, Smith MP, Kane RA (2008) Current techniques in imaging of fistula in ano: three-dimensional endoanal ultrasound and magnetic resonance imaging. Semin Ultrasound CT MR 29:454-71.
11. van Assche G, Dignass A, Reinisch W, et al (2010) European Crohn's and Colitis Organisation (ECCO). J Crohns Colitis 4:63-101.
12. Orsoni P, Barthet M, Portie F, et al. Prospective comparison of endosonography, magnetic resonance imaging and surgical findings in anorectal fistula and abscess complicating Crohn's disease. Br J Surg 1999; 86:360–4.
13. Steele SR, Kumar R, Feingold DL, Rafferty JL, Buie WD; Standards Practice Task Force of the American Society of Colon and Rectal Surgeons (2011) Practice parameters for the management of perianal abscess and fistula-in-ano. Dis Colon Rectum 54:1465-74

Index

The manufacturer's authorised representative in the EU is Springer Nature Customer Service Centre GmbH, Europaplatz 3, 69115 Heidelberg, Germany. If you have any concerns regarding our products, please contact ProductSafety@springernature.com

Printed and bound by CPI Group (UK) Ltd, Croydon, CR0 4YY
15/07/2026
02167623-0002